Planking
For Pizza

A Body Positive Guide to a
Confident, Healthy, Happy You

Jessica Pack

Copyright © 2016 Jessica Pack
Published by Mango Media Inc.

Design: Laura Mejía
Photo Credits: Jessica Pack

For permission requests, please contact the publisher at:
Mango Publishing Group
2850 Douglas Road, 3rd Floor
Coral Gables, FL 33134 USA
info@mango.bz

For special orders, quantity sales, course adoptions and corporate sales,
please email the publisher at sales@mango.bz.

For trade and wholesale sales, please contact Ingram Publisher Services at
customer.service@ingramcontent.com or +1.800.509.4887.

PLANKING FOR PIZZA: *A Body Positive Guide to a Confident,
Healthy, Happy You*

ISBN: 978-1-63353-473-5

Printed in the United States of America

To my dear friend Ashley, you knew me at my worst and accepted me anyway. I would not be where I am today without your support, encouragement, and words of wisdom that guided me into believing in myself. I can never thank you enough for the positive perspective you have placed in my life to help me change my life for the better. To my sister Rachel, for always seeing and believing the best in me even in the times when I was hard to love. For remaining my one constant and being my number one support system through it all. For hiding with me, crying with me, laughing with me, challenging me, and for always loving me as I was and as I am. Love you always, Rae Rae. And to all the women and girls out there fighting and struggling to know, accept, and feel self-value, worth, respect, and love. Remember you are loved, you are valued, you are worthy, you are important, and you are enough as you are today.

"Raw, real, radiant, and rambunctious, Jess delivers an honest and uplifting truth to her past and present."

—Kim

"HOLY CRAP. SO GOOD. I'm in tears reading your story because it is so incredibly raw and real and so relatable. I love how honest and vulnerable you are with sharing your story because so many young women all over the world will be able to relate. I related so much to your chapter on perfectionism and it also shed a new light on feeling empowered by my imperfections. It feels like we are in this together. Thank you for being brave enough to share your story."

—Julie

"Jess is a gifted story-teller and does an amazing job sharing her own life experiences in such a way that they are simultaneously unique yet relatable, and meaningful yet humorous. She captures the transformative quality in everyday, ordinary experiences, and has the ability to help readers come to understand themselves better through her insights."

—Sara

"Jess perfectly depicts the riveting truth behind the self-conscious imperfections of a perfectionist."

– Casey

"This is a story we can all relate to: a journey into the world of positivity and endless possibilities - once you decide to make the commitment to yourself."

– Morgan

"You took me to a dark place where myself and so many other girls have been. Thank you for your honesty and for sharing how you came from that point to the balanced approach you have today."

– Emma

"Change can be an overwhelming and paralyzing thing. Jessica reminds us that the journey to happiness is one of growth and courage – courage to follow your passions, block out fear, and give yourself grace as you continually evolve."

–Emily

"Jess's ability to be so real and vulnerable is a refreshing drink of water in a world plastered with the ideals of perfection. She removes the veil in front of the raw and relatable insecurities we all struggle to deal with behind closed doors. The only reason you will put this inspirational book down is to get up and get active at realizing a more confident and healthy you."

–Ashley

"I was there to witness the hard times as well as the good times when we were young. After Jessica moved to Florida, distance became our pitfall for keeping in touch. That being said, even with the miles between us I have seen how Jessica has grown with self-love and appreciation for who she is as a person. Now, she sees what I have always seen in her as my big sister. I can only imagine the mental strength it took to get to where she is today. She always talked about writing a book and it's amazing to think now it's becoming a reality. I am fortunate to have her as a sister and her fans are lucky to have her as a role model. This book is a giant plank in her life that displays her strength and ability to not falter. I'm proud of all that she has accomplished and can't wait to see the future progress in her life!"

—Rae

"Reading this chapter hit home emotionally for me; I could relate SO much to Jess's struggles with accepting herself and becoming comfortable in her own skin. While I am now much more confident than I was growing up, I often regress back to my old ways of worrying about the scale, my body, my weight, and comparing myself to others. Jess's 30 days with no numbers plan is just what I need to keep me on track and help me remember my own self-worth. Sometimes you need a kind and gentle reminder to love yourself and share love with others, and this book reminds me to do just that. Thank you, Jess!"

—Shannon

"Jessica's journey is honest, real, and uplifting. Whether you are male, female, skinny, or overweight, you *will* find something that you relate to in her story - there is not a person on earth (that I know of) that is completely comfortable in their own skin. The candidness of her writing is much needed in a world that hides behind concealer and Photoshop."

—Sydney

"The moment we understand that our happiness depends on us and is dictated by the way we act and react; that exact moment we're leading our paths to success and plenitude. It's our faith and trust in ourselves that will give us a meaningful and fulfilling life. This is something that we have to really believe once we finally understand it and we must apply it in every aspect of our lives. Then you'll see how happiness unfolds in front of you. Just as Jessica explained, self-improvement comes from the inside and will surely reflect in the outside."

—Paola

"Jess does a great job capturing the woman bad ass-ery that is loving yourself!! In an open, honest, way Jess really relates to every woman who wants to improve their self-esteem. There is sincerity and comfort in that level of vulnerability."

—Sophie

"Jess' words are raw, authentic, and in a unique way- even spiritual. Her life experiences and previous ways of thinking echo with my own life and journey towards self-discovery. Jess reminds us that we are all human, living our lives the best we can, and most importantly- we are not alone in our fears. She urges us to fall in love with our imperfections, believe in who we are, and embrace life's changes head on! That is where the miraculous happens! This book will empower women across the generations! Relatable and real, Jess has left me with goose bumps! "

— Megan

"Written beautifully, you totally painted a picture in my mind in the beginning with your vacations. I love that you are really open and honest about everything and I am sure a lot of girls need to read this. It is not easy being a girl in this day and age."

—Michelle

"Jess's story reminded me that we are never alone in our struggles in this world. As women, and as human beings. So real, honest, beautiful, and relatable!"

—Alena

"What would happen if, instead of worrying about what you had for breakfast, you focused instead on becoming exquisitely comfortable with who you are as a person? Instead of scrutinizing yourself in the mirror, looking for every bump and bulge, you turned your gaze inward?"

— Lisa Turner,
Losing Weight: What's the Point?

Table of Contents

Foreword

by Becca Anderson

What is so winning about Jessica Pack is her regular girl relatability. I believe her when she says, "If I can do it, you can do it!" I hear her when she talks about realizing her dream job was a nightmare. It makes sense when she says it is okay to be embarrassed about going to the gym and to use that energy to have a great workout. I relate when she confesses her jealousy of perfect girls with perfect bodies. I know exactly what she is talking about when she recalls the "mean girls" in high school and how we must leave all "not good enough stuff" behind in our personal journeys. Jess is truly wise beyond her years and more revelatory and honest in her writing than nearly any other book I have read. Jess goes deep with discussion of how to deal with wobbly self-esteem and how create your own compass (literally! She tells you how to do it here) and navigate forward to your personal happy place. Listen when she tells you how useless it is to compare yourself to others. She is absolutely right- you are uniquely you and celebrating what makes you different will up your joy quotient enormously. I urge you to try the practices and journaling ideas Jess created. They are fantastic, thought-provoking and would be a great thing to do with your girlfriends at your next pizza party.

That's right, you heard me - pizza.

Happy travels on your personal fitness journey, beautiful. Please send postcards!

Introduction

Welcome to a Slice of My Life

For as long as I can remember, I have struggled with an overanxious and worrisome mind. It has plagued me with many feelings of doubt, unworthiness, helplessness, harsh insecurity, fear, self-loathing, and at times depression. As much as I would like to say this book is a guide on "how to enjoy exercise while eating what you want and still getting abs," it is more of a "how to learn to love yourself today despite your mind being an awkward, weird, and embarrassing asshole." I share many stories that are serious, raw, and real; these stem from deep-rooted insecurities that took a lot of courage to reveal. I share lighthearted and comical moments as well. However, I will not be sharing about that time I crapped my pants on an airplane or that other time my dad caught a fly with his tongue, because let's be honest, some details of life are meant to remain a mystery.

Maybe you picked up this book because like myself you think pizza is BAE! But, even if you are one of those liars who says you do not like pizza, maybe you were intrigued because you enjoy planking (still a liar though, because who actually enjoys planking?). Or maybe you picked this book up because you like the idea of establishing and maintaining a balanced lifestyle. I hate to disappoint you, but this story is less about how I established balance and a healthy lifestyle and more about actually discovering that I love living and about how I cultivated a healthy mind and happy heart by adopting a body positive attitude.

I cannot promise that you will walk away with a renewed mind and spirit or that this book will change how you view yourself, but please know that is my main goal with this book. If I can touch even one life, or save one woman or girl from her own self-destruction, it will all be worth it. All the time, fears, anxieties, and doubts I had in sharing my story would be worthwhile. I may not have the best or greatest stories to share with you all. Some may even be a bit boring, but I hope the feelings I share with you all will resonate with you. I hope you feel connected to me as just a normal young woman on a journey to self-awareness and love. My stories are true and honest, even the self-deprecation. I sincerely hope you find my negative thoughts to be relatable in some way so that you can begin to question your negative inner dialogue. I want you to be able to change it so that you are able to lay a foundation of hope, change, positivity, happiness, and above all else, self-love and respect.

Without boring you with all the details, my journey to a body-positive mindset began on June 1, 2015. I saw a picture of myself over Memorial Day weekend and was appalled by what I saw. I was in denial about how I had let myself go. Mostly I saw a reflection of a young woman who was lost, lonely, anxiety-ridden, a bit depressed, hopeless, unworthy, and lacking in self-respect and love. I did not recognize myself. I had lost all understanding of my very being.

In all honesty, when I started my fitness Instagram account, I was going to use it to make fun of myself and how I sucked at fitness. I was out of shape and did not know how to exercise or make healthy living a priority. I thought it would be a spectacle to witness and wanted to document all the "fails." I created the Instagram mostly in the hopes to remain accountable to my weight loss goals, but I really did not think my body or mind would make any changes. I have a yo-yo past and thought that was going to be the same scenario for this new lifestyle I was trying to find. But what I found was so much deeper, more powerful, and impactful than I could have ever imagined.

What I found was I love fitness and living a healthy lifestyle. I love finding my power in both my strengths and weaknesses. I love watching myself grow and change. After my time of self-destruction, I needed this new path to rebuild myself and redefine my purpose, passions, and meaning. I found that everything I thought I wanted and who I thought was were actually far from the truth. My fitness undertakings helped me realize that the path I had been on for so many years was in fact the wrong one. I am now at a point where I am ready and willing to walk a new path.

I would say I am currently at a fork in the road in terms of which path to take, except that fork has about 18 prongs.

But that is the beauty in life, if plan A does not work, there is always a new direction we can take. I have fallen in love with living a healthy and active lifestyle, and it has contributed to helping me fall more in love with myself and who I am becoming. Of course, there are still missing pieces and I am trying to build the whole picture. I am not there yet! I now understand how poor body image, low self-esteem, and worthlessness held me back from being in touch with my truest self. Plank by plank, I am overcoming, and I want the same for you.

As I sit here writing this, I question everything about my journey, my story, this book. Can I do this? Can I help women feel better about themselves in their current state? Can I make a difference? Are these the right messages and stories to share? Is my story enough? Am I worthy to share my ordinary story? What will people say? What will people think? As you can see from all these question, my fears and doubts are surfacing as my anxiety takes over. But I have allowed both my heart and soul to take over my mind this time. My mind is telling me NO, but my heart and soul are saying YES to sharing my story because this is where my passion lies. I want to help women and young girls learn that their value and worth is beyond what others say and what their mind says about how their body looks. We put so much emphasis and value into what we look like that we forget to discover who we are. We are SO much more than what our bodies portray and this is the biggest message I want you to walk away with.

My negative thoughts and feelings stem from a rocky childhood filled with too many secrets to count. As much as I want to share every detail of the good and the bad of my childhood, I have left out details from my past to protect those I love. Please understand the insecure feelings and negative thoughts I protected in my mind for so long are very deep-rooted. Part of this whole journey is overcoming these past thoughts and feelings so I can pursue a life I love living. It is this lifestyle that will bring the meaning, connection, and happiness I so desire.

I want to help women feel great and confident in the skin they were given. I want girls to learn how to be happy and confident in the now while pursuing goals and dreams, whether they be body goals or life transformation. I recently took the step of becoming a life coach, because I know my passion in life is to help women and girls feel confident and comfortable in WHO they are and not allowing what they look like to define their worth. I want to help empower and support women to embrace their imperfections, so that they can pursue life with a new mindset and in a healthy and happy manner in the ways that works for them. This is just my story and how I have found a more positive and body confident mindset. There is no guarantee this book will change your perspective about yourself, because ultimately it starts with YOU being ready and willing to make a change. I cannot want it **for** you, you have to want it for yourself. Along the way, I have learned some people think it is others that need to change, and those people are hard to help. You must be willing to look inside and realize your worth, your potential, and your happiness is found within and not through others. This being said, what worked for me is not necessarily or guaranteed to work for anyone else, but I truly believe transformation begins withIN!

I found that by changing my mindset, I still see my imperfections and flaws, yet I no longer feel confined and bound by their existence. I have realized they do not define my being. I am not always content with my body, but I have come to a point where I am more confident and happy with myself than ever before. This mental change did not come from changing my body, it came from changing my mind so that my heart could break barriers and become a little softer and kinder to my whole being. Only by changing my attitude could my authentic self be slowly realized. My soul is finally coming alive, no longer being concealed by my body or wounded by my heart.

I have so many *shoulda-coulda-woulda* moments that I regret. But I have always learned and grown most from my mistakes, rarely have I grown from successes. Maybe I should not have bought a house at age 24. My first job became unbearable, but I had to stick with it, though I would have loved to quit and move back home. However, had that happened, I might not have started a fitness journey. I might not have found the self-love and body confidence I now have. Mostly, I probably would not have gotten to know myself; I might never have realized my fullest potential and deepest passions. Our passions lead us to who we really are. This defines you, not your body. Allow yourself to crumble a bit, allow yourself to fail. Our faults and failures are only PART of our being. My mistakes and what I learned made me stronger. I am not a perfect person; I no longer strive to be. I have learned that my flaws do not define me, yet they are a part of me, and to feel completely whole, I need to accept them. Every day is a new challenge and opportunity to learn something new and discover something different. I learned that changing my mindset helped me with being content with my body as it is today. However, I am still working on exploring, creating, and defining my truest heart and soul. I know that is where my most authentic self hides. I want to bring her out. I want to be all of me all the time. Yet my mental and bodily restrictions inhibit that. My journey has evolved into something far deeper than making fun of myself and how I suck at fitness. I found I actually am capable and stronger than I ever thought possible. Although my body may not yet express the visual signs of strengths I have envisioned in my mind, I know I am fitter, happier, and healthier than ever before. I proved myself wrong and I continue to do so daily.

This is just my own journey. A few of my past and present experiences, snapshots of my story. It is unique to me. But if you can resonate with anything I say and feel a little better about yourself and begin to question and change your inner dialogue, then all my fears and doubts about sharing my story will be worthwhile. I am often told that I am "so brave and vulnerable" for being open with my feelings and insecurities. I always tell my friends that I do not feel brave. The feedback helps me understand the courage involved in my willingness to go to a place many people are afraid to go. I don't like sharing my rawest feelings, but I am willing to feel the pain. Embracing the discomfort is worth it so that I can move forward and heal. Sharing all this is helpful, too, after keeping it to myself for so long. Knowing I am not alone and sharing my deepest insecurities helps me to not just begin my healing, but to begin to be more in touch with my most authentic truth. I think many of us tend to struggle alone in our dark moments and anything that seems to be a bit "emotionally unstable" is instantly judged.

We are raised to believe we must always put out our best front forward; showing any self-doubt is a sign of weakness. No one wants to admit they are struggling and suffering, but it's not like we planned life to be that way. It's not intentional. I have yet to meet a person who genuinely enjoys self-destruction. I tended to numb and hide from that pain instead of just sitting with it, truly feeling all of it and letting it absorb. Facing that pain head on is a means to destroy the demons inside that don't belong. There are so many whose stories are similar to mine. This is a reality that I know MANY if not all women share. And my greatest hope in sharing my story is that you know you are not alone in your insecurities or struggles. Like seedlings, as we begin to understand our truths and allow self-love in, we need the darkness to guide us to the light in order to bloom. What you plant now, you harvest later. Both a dandelion and an oak tree start in the darkness as seeds. You can choose to be flimsy and blow away easily at the slightest of winds, or you can choose to grow strong, tall, and unbreakable. Do not plant that weed of self-doubt in your mind because it will simply overtake and destroy your body, heart, and soul. Plant positivity in your mind, so that you can establish strong roots and grow in strength from the inside to the out.

So, cheers babes to living life with a healthy mind, positive heart,

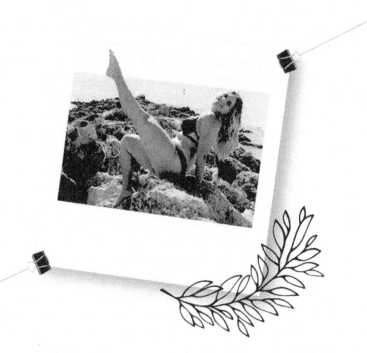

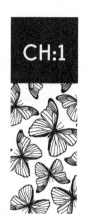

Fall In Love With Your Selfie

I hesitantly walk towards the back of the boat, staring into the murky water below. I scan the edges of the shoreline. I am in the midst of an anxiety dilemma. Was I going to choose fear or choose comfort? I had witnessed the sweet manatees' little faces when they breached for air moments before deciding to get into the water. I turn to our tour guide needing to know but not wanting to ask the most important question, the one no one else seemed to be concerned about, "So... are there alligators in this water?"

He gingerly laughs and replies, "Well, I have been doing this for a few years now and have only ever seen two. But it is a river, and we are in Florida. Chances are pretty high that there are in fact alligators, but you most likely will not see them."

"Great, how comforting," I silently told myself. However, I knew the manatees were near! The group had to quietly and calmly get into the dark, frigid waters. I decided to go for it and very slowly slipped down into the river. Fear consumed me. I started hyperventilating through the snorkel. I was terrified. I swam over to where the group had congregated and placed my face in the water to look around. Nothing. All this fear, anxiety, and panic, and there was nothing to be seen except cloudiness. We floated in the cold waters for several minutes, looking around for the manatees. Suddenly, out of nowhere, two giant gray masses appeared. They were so close I could touch them, but I backed away from them, too taken aback by their gargantuan size. That was more enough excitement for me; I was ready to get back in the boat. But the group followed them and I carefully swam along.

We tracked this pair of manatees for a few minutes. They would dive out of site and then suddenly reappear out of the opaque waters. I could not help but fear that the next time an animal came out of nowhere it would be an alligator, or some creepily gigantic fish. Thankfully, all we saw were the manatees. Our tour guide said we had been following them long enough and that it was time to head to another spot. I had had my fun and was doubtful about getting in the water again. But when the guide said the next spot was a mother manatee and her calf were, I was suckered in all over again. It was extra exciting to share this rare experience with my friend, who had come to town just to see me.

We arrived at the next spot and thankfully it was much shallower water, so we could walk and didn't have to dive in and swim in the unknown murk. But as it turned out, walking was not allowed, so that the surrounding sediment wouldn't be disturbed. I immediately noticed three other boats and a mass of people clustered in one spot. We had to wait for a few boats to clear so we could get out and see the manatees. Sure enough, lying in silence on the shore, there was my biggest nightmare - a giant effing alligator! Okay, maybe not actually a giant. It was a youngster of less than four feet long, but still long enough to put me on edge. The alligator was simply sunbathing on the water's edge, but it was too close for my comfort.

The time had come to get into the water, but I was filled with trepidation. My friend persuaded me to get in. The water was muddy and filled with sediment due to people stirring it up. It felt like we were in the water for eons, but I only saw the manatees briefly. I was ready to be done. When we finally headed back to the boat, I noticed the alligator was gone. Luckily, we survived and headed back to the dock. When we got back to the main office, my friend wanted to take a picture in front of the sign to remember this special experience. It took some convincing, but I finally agreed; I did not usuallytake pictures of myself. That day, May 24, 2015, would forever be a day of significance for me. In a way, it became a renaissance of my soul. The hours that followed that exciting and eventful morning changed my life forever.

My friend's cat allergies meant she had to stay in a hotel since my tiny house has two cats. I dropped her off at her hotel and returned home, ready to crash. Before nodding, off I saw the notification: "Your friend has tagged you in a photo on Facebook." Instant dread set in. I remained calm at first, hoping it was the cute snorkeling selfie we had taken in the water, but what I saw shocked me.

Glumly, I said to my roommate, "Oh my gosh. Look at this terrible photo I was just tagged in. I look awful. Seriously, I look like a freaking beached whale! Am I really this big?"

My roommate calmly and with a bit of an eye roll replied, "Let me see." Slight pause. "You absolutely do not look like a beached whale. You just do not see yourself the way the rest of the world sees you."

It was in that moment, that one second of time, that I truly allowed myself to absorb the meaning of that statement. After a moment of reflection, it finally clicked. For once I saw myself with my heart, not my mind. In that moment, I decided I was done with self-sabotage. I was tired of being critical and hard on myself. I was over the self-hate and disrespect. I was finished with feeling unlovable, unworthy, talentless, undesired, lonely, incomplete, and not good or pretty enough. I decided I was worthy of feeling loved, being enough as I am, and deserving of happiness. This was the day I chose self-love.

My morning ritual and mantra always stemmed from a place of negativity. I would say things to myself like, "You look gross today. Your thighs are disgusting. Why are you so fat? Why can't you lose the weight? You would be pretty and lovable if you just would lose the weight." It was this unkindness, bitterness, and lack of self-respect that I was so fed up with. Why was it just so hard to love myself? Why did I let my bodily expression define my existence so much? And mostly, why was I afraid to truly see myself?

I had always thought that the only way I would truly be content and happy with myself was if I lost weight. This time, however, something was different. My goals and mindset had changed. Yes, I wanted to lose weight and get into shape, but what I wanted more was a state of health and happiness. I had created all this sadness, loneliness, and despair, never realizing just how much my negative mindset about my body had impacted every aspect of my life. I had mentally and emotionally built walls to guard my heart and created obstacles to safeguard my soul from truly being treasured. I went about life wanting to remain invisible, but for once, I was ready for my heart and soul to be seen.

I spent the next week creating a game plan. The next Monday was the first day of June, and it seemed like the perfect time to start a new routine. I had been following a 12 week program on Instagram for several months prior. I thought, "What is 12 weeks in a lifetime? It is nothing! I owe that time to myself to try to be a healthier, better, happier me." Yet there was still a lot of fear and doubt that this time would be just like all the other times. I was worried that it might just be a fad that would only last a few days, maybe a couple of weeks, before I gave up, threw in the towel, and went back to my sad and miserable ways.

The first two weeks were incredibly challenging. I did not follow the program strictly. I figured anything was better than nothing, but I did not want to simply half-ass it and do the bare minimum. I knew in order for it to be effective, I had to follow the guide more stringently. Two weeks into my new life plan, I took a huge leap of faith: I created my fitness Instagram. Taking those first few progress photos just validated the reasons why I was doing this. In the midst of judging, criticizing, and ridiculing every part of my body, something monumental happened: I stopped myself. I knew that harsh and pessimistic thoughts would not yield positive results. Instead of ridiculing my body, I changed my mindset and gently reminded myself that I was at last working on being the best that I could be. I just needed a lot of patience, a little kindness, and most of all acceptance of myself in that present moment. My journey was only just beginning.

I knew it would take more than 12 weeks going into this new program to produce what I envisioned as my "goal" body. I was roughly eight weeks into the program when I started noticing progress. I was not only taking weekly progress pictures of myself, but posting more selfies in general. I had never taken so many pictures of myself! Something profound was occurring. Yes, I was happy with the physical changes I was noticing, but I also started seeing myself beyond my physical body. I began to see a growing confidence. I started to see my smile growing brighter. I started to see genuine happiness emerging. I started to see the true me.

For the longest time, I had avoided both mirrors and photos. Mirrors had become temporary moments of negativity, whereas photos made a more impactful impression because I could analyze and truly see the emotions behind my false expression and pick apart flaws. I avoided mirrors except to apply makeup. I did not want to see my body and did everything in my power to avoid seeing myself naked in a mirror. I had always placed my worth in my body, and since I did not have a "perfect" body, I judged that I was simply not worthy of the things I desired. By avoiding photos, I was choosing not to see myself; but in doing so, I was failing to truly experience the moment and make lasting memories. I began to miss being present in the moment, because I was allowing my body insecurities to control my ability to simply be.

The happiness I was seeking was not in the physical changes I was making. It was much deeper. The happiness I began to find was the recognition that I was not simply defined by my external being. My happiness came from realizing all of who I was and what I was meant to become. I had spent my whole life seeking happiness by changing my physical body. Although the physical progress I was making contributed to my growing confidence and happiness, I realized that my worth and feelings of being enough were not found in my body shape or size. They were found in understanding my truest potential and all that I was meant to become.

By taking photos of myself regularly to document my journey, I began to realize that I was so much more than my body. My bodily flaws were no longer defining me. I had used my fat rolls, arm jiggle, cellulite, and pimples as excuses to not be seen. I thought my worth and value resided in my outward physicality. I did not feel like the 'cute girl', and I never felt beautiful. I saw myself as fat and unattractive and used these critical words to describe myself. My perspective on my body only began to shift several months into my journey. It did not happen overnight; it happened over time. I realized that the happiness I was seeking did not stem from the desire to change my body, it came from finding and realizing my true worth. And I saw that my worth, value and enough-ness has nothing to do with my body but everything to do with my being. I began to truly see for the first time that I was not fat, I had fat. Maybe I did not always feel beautiful, but I was beautiful because beauty truly is internal. For me, beauty is not found in our bodies; it is in our hearts, minds, and souls.

As I began for the first time to see myself, and not my body, my negative thoughts started to dissolve. I saw happiness and a growing confidence in my pictures, and I FELT it too. I used to take at least 30 pictures trying to get the "right" one, but as my perspective changed, I found I was taking fewer and fewer pictures and was content with all of them. Because I wasn't looking for or at my flaws, I was looking at me. And I was no longer afraid to share the "ugly" because I did not allow that to define myself. I became content in who I was, defects and all. Amazingly, other people never saw the flaws I would point at or pick apart. They complimented the unseen. And by others recognizing the unseen, I was able to step out of the notion of seeing my body, and truly see myself through the eyes of others.

My growing body positivity stemmed from not what I was seeing, but from what was unseen. All of these revelations took time. But it all happened because I learned to fall in love with my selfie. I began to compliment myself. But not in a "*Dayum* girl, you are looking fine today" kind of way. I complimented who I was becoming. I complimented my kindness. I complemented my compassion. I complimented my strength. I even complimented my weakness. I complimented my determination. I complimented my courage. I complimented my vulnerability. Some days I complimented my looks, but most days I chose to compliment my inner traits, because I had finally learned to separate my body and appearances from my worth.

June 1, 2015, was the day I chose self-betterment. I found my superpower that day. This power is the ability to choose. The best thing about this superpower is that it is not mine alone. You have the power to choose too. You make millions of choices in your lifetime, but it is the tiny decisions you make each and every day that add up to change. You have the power, the ability, and the freedom to make a change, too. You can choose to snooze a little longer, or wake up a little earlier for a morning mediation or self-development session. You can choose to eat the salad you have prepared for lunch or go out with coworkers for pizza. You can choose to hit the gym or be a little lazy. You can choose to live in a body you're not comfortable with or you can choose to change it. You can choose to love yourself or hate yourself. That power is yours, and no one can take that away from you. There may be people who try, no doubt, but you have the ability to choose to let their negativity define you and bring you down or to become stronger by knowing your worth stems from a source far deeper than your body. You, too, can choose to love yourself and your selfie!

Selfie Project

I have never said, "Will you take my picture?" more than I have since I began my fitness journey. In a way, I am sure I have felt compelled to take pictures simply to document my quest. But the fact that I tend to choose self-images over food or other images speaks to the positive self-reflections I have developed. In the past, I would grudgingly agree to take a picture but would request that the picture always be from the waist up. I never wanted really anything below my chest to be seen. In the time I have spent on bettering myself, I have learned that is it not what my body looks like that defines the image. I have learned to look beyond my body and see the moment itself. For me, photos are now not about wearing the fanciest of clothes or what my hair looks like or having the best professional pictures. It is so much more than that. It is about the warmth, the shared moment, the laughter, the expressions, the people I am with – the love, the bonds, the hugs, the happiness, the sadness, the emotions captured on film. Pictures capture connection, and for me, connection is how I pursue a meaningful life. Looking back, I am so sad that I spent more time behind a camera than in front of it capturing memories with those I shared experiences with. I lost the moments and, in a way, the memory of the experience. By not being present in images, it was almost like I was disconnecting from my existence by intentionally not being seen. Now, instead of looking at it as "missed life," I am so thankful for the clarity I have found, to be able to look beyond imperfections and truly love and live life without ideas about my body hindering me anymore.

I look back on old pictures I have taken and cannot help but feel regret for the sadness I often expressed in photos. Often I was in beautiful locations on a wonderful adventure, yet I looked so unhappy to be there. And truly, this unhappiness stemmed from the unhappiness I felt with myself. I now experience this as joy in the moment; as I have learned to find contentment and acceptance of myself in photos, I see the beauty of life itself.

Selfie-Acceptance Starts With YOU

I challenge you all to a little project of learning to love your selfie. Like me, you might not necessarily love this photo project at first. But you must begin with acceptance of your present state and realizing that your worth is not based simply on your external expression. It is so easy to judge, ridicule, and see the things we do not like about our photos first. It is much harder to see yourself as others do

Our hearts, our minds, our souls are what should be valued, the significance of what we contribute to society. Our bodies are what allow us to live and do the things we love to do; however, it is what lies inside that defines our being. A few fat rolls, acne, or cellulite has absolutely no place in creating the value of your WHO. WHO you are matters. WHAT you look like does not, thoughcertainly, you don't show up to a big job interview looking like a slob. I am shy by nature. Always have been. But I am so beyond ready for my soul to break through my shell. I easily turn to comfort and safety like a turtle instead of battling the uncomfortable head on. But growth only comes out of stepping out of that shell. I want to ask you to do a little personal development project to fall in love with your selfie and hopefully begin to start stepping out of your shell of body negativity.

The following are techniques and exercises I have harvested along my fitness journey. Whenever I found myself being self-critical, I would redirect my thoughts. If I caught myself saying self-sabotaging things like, "Gosh your love handles are just so gross and noticeable today. Eat and do better so you can get rid of these flabby things." I would then redirect my thoughts to something like, "Ok, stop it. Maybe you have love handles. But it is ok. Today you are going to the gym later and eating right so that one day they will be less visible. But you may always have them, so accept them as they are today. A part of your being! Besides, you are still shining because you are committed to making yourself a better you!" I cannot promise you will find self-love through this exercise, but my hope is maybe you can begin to redirect your thoughts in a more loving manner. Below are a few photo prompts that I hope will help you create a more positive attitude towards yourself in photos. These should be done when you feel like challenging yourself. Don't force it, simply allow yourself to feel it when you are ready!

Body Positive Photo Prompts:

○ Take a picture in something you're uncomfortable in. It could be anything for you. Maybe it is a bathing suit or crop top or shorts, the point is to feel a little discomfort. This can be done in the security of your own home.

○ Take a picture in something you love wearing. It should be something you feel great in!

○ In a fearless moment, ask a friend, or a stranger if you are feeling brave, to take a photo of you doing something you feel truly represents you.

○ It is difficult to capture a vulnerable moment because most people do not want to open themselves up to feeling exposed; however, if there is something that makes you feel vulnerable, capture that moment as best as you can. It could be as simple as lying by the pool in a bikini when you feel you are not "bikini ready" (– a totally BS concept. BTW, I can guarantee you are bikini ready today! Own it girl!)

◦ What do you absolutely love doing? Being artistic? Athletic? Surrounded by loved ones? Take a photo of yourself doing that thing you love to do.

Now ask yourself the following questions based on the pictures above:

What do you see in this image? What do you feel?

Is what you see negative? Are you seeing yourself for your physical flaws? If so, negate that negative thought with something optimistic. Ideally, negate it with something positive that is not about your physical expression.

Do you like what you see? Do you love it? How do you honestly feel about it?

Remember not to seek out the things you dislike intentionally, because that tends to create a direction of looking for the imperfections. If you find yourself looking for weaknesses and only seeing the negative and things you do not like, ask what is it you are truly looking for in yourself? If it is some sort of internal peace or balance, I know you will start speaking more compassionately about yourself. Repeat these prompts, or create your own unique ones, until your inner conversation changes. Soon enough, you will fall in love with your selfie, because you are not looking just at what is, but hopefully at the whole picture. Life is beautiful, babe, and so are you!

If you feel brave enough to share and own your selfie, feel free to share on Instagram using hashtag #pizzaplankselfieproject and tag me in your photos so I can see them!

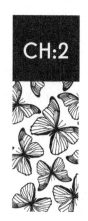

Fit AF?

CH:2

Prior to committing to a healthy lifestyle, I would have definitely called myself a "yo-yo" dieter. In high school, I found myself restricting. I never was diagnosed with or considered myself to have an eating disorder, but I definitely limited calories and would be really upset with myself if I went over by even 5 calories. It would come and go in phases. I had always heard 1200 calories was the lowest "healthy" daily limit, so at times I would restrict myself to that calorie limit. I would stick to this calorie goal for a few weeks or months at a time, then I would realize that the calorie restriction was not yielding results fast enough, and I would findmyself frustrated and give up, because I liked food for comfort.

During my "off" months in high school, I would often get home from school and cram anything and everything in sight into my mouth before my mom got home. Most of the time it was unhealthy things like chips, pretzels, and cheese crackers. From what I can remember, this is when my binge eating habits began. I did not feel "allowed" to eat junk food in the amounts I wanted to, so I always felt the need to get a junk food "fix" in secret. Since I was the first home usually, I would quickly throw my stuff down and head to the pantry first. I would grab whatever I was craving and eat as fast as I could by a window, watching and waiting for my mom to come home so she would not see that I was snacking. Obviously, she could see that contents of the bags were decreasing, so she would ask me whether or not I was eating the snack foods. I always blamed my sister, but I think my mom knew better.

Growing up with divorcehad many challenges, one of which was that my parents differed drastically on eating habits. My dad pretty much allowed my sister and me to eat anything and everything we wanted, whereas my mom tended to limit us. We usually could only have a suggested-serving portion of what we desired with our mom, rather than, say, a whole sleeve of cookies at my dad's house. (He would limit us if it got out of hand, but most of the time he was more lenient and flexible.) When I got to college, binging became far easier. I did not feel the need to hide. I could do so quietly or comfortably in my own room. I tried my best to eat healthy, but it was really challenging, especially when I was on the meal plan. Even then, I tried to have a stash of snacks in my room at all times. As a college student who stayed up late most nights, snacks were essential. We also had a dining hall on campus that was open 24 hours on weekdays where I often went with friends to consume large amounts of food at midnight. It was fun, and nobody was judging me.

I didn't rebel in college by going out and partying, I rebelled by eating. I began to notice all the binging starting to catch up with me. I was in denial about not just my weight gain, but weight in general. I always thought I was maintaining roughly a 130 pound number, when in reality I probably had crept up to the 150 pound range. Although I would walk most places on campus, I was still rather sedentary. I would occasionally go to the gym with a friend, but it was never anything consistent. My "yo-yo" life then was always one of binging and restricting. I never found a happy or healthy balance.

In 2011, I started to really notice my weight gain and began to feel even more down on myself. I realized I needed to do something a bit drastic to hopefully help me break my binge cycle and signed up for a sprint triathlon. I had several months to plan and prepare, but did very little training for the event itself, #typical. I practiced for the swimming portion the most, as that was the part I was most comfortable doing. I biked the course once and went on a few long bike rides with my mom. I ran very little because running is just not my thing. The event day approached far more quickly than I expected, but I was committed and had no choice but to stick it out and do my best. Unsurprisingly, swimming was the easiest leg for me, but I really struggled during the bike and running portions. Regardless, I still completed it. I held onto that sense of accomplishment, because although I was not in shape nor at a desired weight, I had set my mind to complete a triathlon and did not let these things hold me back.

Deep down, I knew if I had trained more or been in better shape, the race would have been easier for me. My hope had been that I would train for this event, get into shape, love doing a triathlon, and continue with an exercise routine after the race. But it did not quite work that way. Several months later, I had not stepped foot inside a gym except when forced. In the spring semester of 2012, I signed up for P.E. because it was required, but it ended up being a great decision for me. I established a great routine and ended up losing 20 pounds by the end of the semester. But sometimes those things don't last.

More Marathons

I moved to Florida a few years ago. Being alone in a new state made it easy for binging habits to pick up full force again. I do not know how much I weighed when I moved to Florida, but I assume that from the time I moved to Florida to when I started my fitness routine, I probably gained anywhere from 10-20 pounds. Eating whole pizzas and family-sized bags of chips in one sitting became routine for me. I knew I had to change.

The best way I knew how to break a cycle was to once again sign up for a big event for which I was not at all in shape. I had heard about the Disney Princess Half Marathon and thought it sounded like a lot of fun! Why I thought a running event sounded fun beats me, but I liked the idea of getting to dress up for the event. I had seven months to train and get into shape for it. It truly was the perfect amount of time to establish a workout routine and drop some needed pounds. However, December rolled around too quickly; two months before the half marathon, and I had not run even once. I started panicking, wondering how can I ever run a half marathon when I cannot even run a mile? So I started forcing myself into the gym. But by the time of the event, I was only up to a five mile run.

Then it was race day again and I had no choice. I was committed. My family also signed up to do it with me, so they were in town, and I could not let them down. My parents are runners and my sister was a bit more active than I was at the time, so I knew they would not stay behind with me. For a while, my sister stayed back with me, but my parents bolted ahead. They are not fans of crowds and this was one crowded event! Soon I became too slow for my sister too, so she jogged ahead. I am not sure if the pace I was maintaining could even be considered a "jog", but I was still "jogging" in my mind. It might have been as slow as a turtle in molasses, but I. Was. Jogging.

The excitement around me honestly fueled me to keep going. I was definitely feeling tired and was ready for it to be over, but I had a long way to go. I ended up making it to mile 8.5 at a slow jogging pace and took a longer water break there and grabbed one of those Gatorade energy gel things as I was a bit hungry. We had had to wake up at 4:00 a.m. to get to the race, and food was the last thing on my mind that early in the morning. But it was now roughly 8:00 a.m. and I was hungry, and I knew I needed to fuel up. I slowed to a walking pace to rest for a minute before picking back up to a jog.

When I tried jogging again, I simply could not. The pain that had begun to set in my legs was like no other. The immense soreness that had already begun to settle in was quite surprising. I tried and tried again to pick up my sloth's pace jog, but it was too much by this point. I ended up walking the rest of the way with spurts of jogging in between, but I didn't get upset. I hadn't trained, yet I just jogged 8.5 miles. AND I finished all 13.1 miles. This was a huge accomplishment for me and I couldn't help but be proud of myself.

My family wasn't able to stay after the race because they had an eight drive back home. I went home alone and heated a frozen pizza. I ate the whole thing in one sitting and didn't get up from my couch the rest of the day. But hey, I earned that pizza, right? The soreness I felt the remainder of the day and for several days following was unreal. I honestly love feeling sore after a major workout; I was feeling great! Somehow, I continued the habit of no workouts and whole pizzas for the next several months.

My half marathon was in late February, and I began my fitness journey three months later in June. I know this phase helped spark my desire to start working out more regularly, but it didn't happen right away. I was happy I had successfully completed the race, but felt a lingering feeling of disappointment that I had not trained enough to feel more in shape. I was caught up in the comfort of accomplishment. These triathlons and marathons were much like my yo-yo eating habits, a way of compensating with an extreme attempt at exercising. What has been far more rewarding for me since my half marathon has been the little accomplishments each day since my half marathon. Sure, I feel a sense of pride when I complete a half marathon or triathlon, but I now know that nothing compares to the satisfaction of living a healthy lifestyle each and every day. I still have splurging moments, but I try harder and I care more. From the beginning, my main goal has always been

to establish a healthy lifestyle. Despite the occasional
moments of doubt, I am far healthier and happier overall.

What I have learned from these experiences is that one
major event like a half marathon or triathlon will not
suddenly make you healthy, just like eating a piece of
pizza (or a whole one for that matter) will not make you
unhealthy. There will always be an ebb and flow to a
healthy lifestyle. The most important thing is balance. When
slipups occur, and they *will* occur because we are human,
the most important concept I have learned so far is to
simply forgive and forget.

I learned that the more I forgive myself for the lapses, the
more successes I have in the long run. By acknowledging
I slipped up and trying to understand why, I have found
it easier to forget these moments and simply move on.
Binging is a part of my past that no longer defines me. I
have moments when these old habits resurface, but I just
admit to myself that it happened. Then, I move on and try
to do better the next day. A healthy lifestyle is just that, it
is LIFE long. It should be integrated as a part of your life.
Not some fad or quick fix. There will be days when working
out is the last thing on your mind and there will be times
when pizza is the only food that sounds appetizing. That is
perfectly fine. Life is too freaking short to not have a lazy
and relaxing day once in a while. Life is definitely too short
to be completely free of pizza.

Be a #goalgetter not a yo-yoer

I have had lots of therapy in my life, but that doesn't qualify me as a therapist. I can't tell you how to stop an unhealthy eating cycle like mine, because I still experience it myself. All I can really provide here is what has helped me control and deal with my eating habits. But if you are caught in a yo-yo phase, I want you to know you are not alone and there is hope. Lasting and effective change requires patience, consistency, determination, and education. You'll need to understand and accept that it is going to take time and energy to find what works best for you. Real change often requires reaching out and asking for help; this is a very good thing. None of us have all the answers. You don't have to have it all figured out before starting. The beauty of the journey is the evolution of the process and how you evolve as you learn more about yourself and what you are capable of achieving.

How do you break the yo-yo lifestyle? That is the challenge. How do you get to the point where something just "clicks" and works for the long haul? I don't have the magic secret to that. I just knew I had to have 100% confidence and faith in myself when I sought to try something new in the hopes of establishing a healthier lifestyle. Just trust the process and know that lapses and mistakes will happen. When binge moments occur, I never counter it with a restrictive cycle. I acknowledge it, then get right back on track the next day. There are a few questions I have learned to ask myself when a binge episode occurs. These moments tend to occur from a need to numb or feed an emotional feeling or behavior. Whenever I suspect I may be eating out of emotions, I question my poor food choices and what emotions are involved. I have said that I have weak willpower when it comes to overeating. I posted this once on my Instagram, and a follower commented, "Stop saying you have no willpower!!" At first I was really bothered by this. She does not know me and my struggles; how dare she say that? Once I thought about it, I realized I was using lack of willpower as an excuse and an easy way out so I didn't have to understand or feel the emotion fueling the need to binge.

You should always ask yourself if you binged out of hunger. Sometimes I would binge because I did not realize I was just so hungry. And because of that hunger, I over-ate because it was a reaction to feeling that I needed to refuel quickly. Sometimes it would happen because I would go to the grocery store right after the gym and end up buying and eating all of Aisle One within ten minutes. Other times it would happen because I was so busy that I wouldn't get around to eating my first meal until after 3:00 p.m. or later. (I would never advise doing this, I'm just being honest about the good and bad of my journey. I do my best to avoid doing this, but it does happen from time to time.) When this happened, I would go to the store and end up buying enough food for a family of five and eating it all myself. I do not advocate counting calories or macronutrients simply because that works very differently for everyone. Some people have seen incredible success with doing both. I tended to binge more while counting macros, because although it is technically "flexible dieting," I felt restricted. I do plug my food into My Fitness Pal simply to get a baseline understanding of where I fall in both calories and macronutrients. It does help me to have that visual perspective but I try to not get obsessive about it. I say it is worth giving it a try if you think it will work for you. Just remember to try to avoid becoming too obsessive and critical of yourself if you do not hit your goals exactly. Selfie-love!

I know I am not alone in my binge-and-restrict habits of the past. I continue to have the occasional binge mishap. I am not perfect and never will be. Guess what, that's okay! If you mess up, check in, forgive and move on. What helped me overcome my yo-yo past was to stick to about an 80% healthy and clean food to 20% processed food lifestyle. When a binge episode occurs, I never counter it with restriction or avoidance. I simply get right back on track. If that sounds easier said than done, the other part I learned is to forgive and forget. What I really mean by forgive is to not to forgive the act of indulging, but to forgive yourself for any harsh or unkind words you may put upon yourself. I have said terrible things to myself after a slipup, and it only makes me feel worse. I simply forgive myself for allowing the unkind words or actions to have taken place and move on,both for yourself and to be able to live a healthy lifestyle. It takes commitment above everything. Commit to breaking your yo-yo habits. Commit to working out every day, even if it is a ten minute walk. Commit to YOU. You deserve it. There are *so* many people out there who have done it, you should not be any different. You can break the cycle, it just begins with a little self-discovery and tapping into your truest potential.

How can you in turn become a **#goalgetter**? For me, this came from changing my attitude and my outlook as I approached this lifestyle change. In the past, I was motivated by wanting to be skinnier so I would feel more attractive. The problem with this is that it is an internally-driven, deeply negative type of motivation. When I switched from weight loss as my sole measure of worth to knowing I was already worthy is when health and happiness became my main objectives. Only then did the motivation stick. Now, when I set goals, I try not to set up myself up for failure by trying to tackle all my goals at once. Each month, I set new goals for just one month. At times I get anxious about everything I want to accomplish and end up making a list of 10+ goals to achieve in one month's time. All that does is bog me down with trying to multitask and do everything at once so I end up not actually accomplishing anything. I have worked hard at changing my thought process around this; I simply focus on one goal each month. Truth be told, I set two goals a month. I set one goal that is fitness-related and one goal that is life-related. I find this makes it far more manageable and easier to stay on task. For example, one of my fitness goals was to focus on fat loss for one month. Instead of thinking of all the ways I could target that goal, I simply said I would add in 30 minutes of cardio a day on top of my routine. Just for one month. After that, I would assess how it worked and if I *felt* any difference. It truly takes time and effort to know if something is going to work for you. Instead of trying to do everything at once, there are a few ways you can refocus, so you set goals that are actually achievable.

Be a #goalgetter:

- First, you need to have realistic expectations. What is a realistic goal for you? Say you want to lose 20 pounds in one month for that special event? Try again! Quick solutions will never yield life-long results.

- What is one thing I can do differently today?

- What is one thing I can do differently this week?

- What is one thing I can do differently this month?

- What are my three BIG goals I want to accomplish this year?

- Set goals that are action-based, not results-driven. If you focus too much on the end result, you lose the actual strategic foundation you can use to work toward an end result. The result will never occur without the action and plan set in place. How can you rework your goals so that they are driven by a measurable control?

There are a few things to be mindful of when setting fitness-related goals. Your body may never look the way your mind wants it to; simply put, there is no way of knowing what you will look like until you get there. Even when you get there, you may not like or be happy with what you see. That is why it is so important to learn to be content in the now. This will even help you with currentinsecurities while you are working towards the things you wish to accomplish. It also makes your "final product" far more rewarding. You will have a greater sense of accomplishment and pride if you love yourself every step of the way. Remember, this is not about achieving a "perfect" body. It should be about the process of learning to respect and treat your body with care while crafting a confident mind so that your soul can prosper.

When setting lifestyle or passion-driven goals, remember to make sure they are yours and yours alone. It is so very easy to want to live someone else's life or have what they have. You cannot live anyone else's life, as you would not be living YOUR truth. However, you CAN CREATE a life you want to live and love. Why do we get so involved with other's lives that we forget to live our own beautiful life? What does your dream life look like? Now, how will you accomplish your vision? Remember, think process, not product. Perhaps you feel stuck because you do not have the right opportunities, or support, or funding to chase those dreams of yours. You have the power to create the opportunity and make it happen. You just need a little faith in the process of taking some risks to pursue a life you love.

FOMO

Growing up, I was always a painfully shy, anxious, and worrisome child. At some level, I am still this way as an adult. There are certain social situations that paralyze me with fear of embarrassment; I am hesitant to be openly vulnerable. I still worry about things that are out of my control, and I am seeing a therapist so I can learn to cope with my anxiety. It is easy for my apprehension to get the best of me and allow negative thoughts to flood my mind. I have learned to manage all this slowly but surely. It begins with fear and facing it head on. If I can do it, you can do it, for certain.

Throughout grade school, I was relatively smart. I felt it was my job to excel in school so that I could get into a good college. Although I often knew the answers, I wouldn't make eye contact with the teacher to avoid being called on to say them out loud. I was afraid of having the wrong answer or mispronouncing the words while reading a passage from a chapter. For me, those things showed weakness, which in turn resulted in humiliation. I did not want to appear weak, because I always had to be so strong, given the many things I was dealing with in my family. I did not want to feel mortified, because somehow as a young girl, embarrassment translated into a strange sense of insignificance. I always felt extremely self-conscious. Just being recognized or noticed when I was called on in class brought on a feeling of shame, as if I was unworthy of being seen. My face would glow a crimson red, and I am sure the heat my body produced would have been enough to melt chocolate. As much as I tried, I could not control these reactions.

This all stemmed from my shyness no doubt, but the anxiety consumed me to the point of not even putting myself out there. For a child, I worried about a lot of things. I would worry about the most insignificant things. I wonder at times if worrying is a genetically inherited trait, because my paternal grandma is the queen of worrying. I know much of the anxiety came from my family home. It is difficult to tackle such ingrained emotions at a young age when it is nearly impossible to see how these things can consume and control your future. There is much value in maturing and growing older. I still worry about the silliest of things and can be really shy, but I no longer let fear and embarrassment consume me, Embarrassment shows my human side. Somehow I came up with the idea that I was not allowed to be "human" and had to be so perfect all the time. I have learned to truly allow myself to let go and laugh at the things that are human about me, because I have found out that I value and love that side of myself the most.

Fear can be very consuming in our lives. It can overtake and paralyze us to the point where we feel that we are missing out because we allow it to hold us back. But when we face our fears, that is when enchantment happens. That is when transformation occurs. Facing one's fears may not have a positive outcome every time, but when embarrassment happens, that is when growth takes place. And there is a positive to growth. It may be a bit painful at first, but there is always merit to reflecting on the embarrassment and understanding why facing the fear failed. For me, facing fears always yields some sort of positive despite how mentally challenging it may seem.

I was always been afraid to actually commit to changing my lifestyle because I feared my results would never be "enough." I thought that maybe I would reach the level of "skinny" I wanted to achieve and that I still would not find myself attractive enough or worthy or deserving of being admired for what and who I am. Fear has held me back in so many ways. I got to the point where I was so ashamed of how I viewed myself that the fear was worth facing.

My fears have not always been focused on my body specifically, but on my whole being in general. I cannot really remember a time when I was afraid to do something because I was embarrassed by my body. If it involved wearing a bathing suit, I would go ahead, but that doesn't mean I would do it without discomfort. I have never been a fan of wearing shorts, but if it was really hot outside, I would. Although I wouldn't hide or simply not go to the event because it required a bathing suit or shorts, I still would analyze and pick everything apart. Despite my physical insecurities, though, my biggest fear was participation and connection with others. If there were only a few of my friends present and the rest were strangers, I would be uncomfortable and shy. Or if it was an event with all strangers, I would more than likely not even go. I would be afraid of saying the wrong thing or doing something embarrassing. I was mostly afraid of not being liked for who I am.

As I have grown older and have discovered myself a bit more through my fitness journey, I have realized how irrational and ridiculous some of my fears have been. Yes, it is unpleasant when someone doesn't like you, but I have accepted it is okay. Not everyone will. I have learned to separate my physicality from how people view me. Sharing a fitness journey online makes you susceptible to criticism and ridicule. I have seen some very ugly comments on other people's photos and have been victim to these online bullies myself. But comments like "fat" or "ugly" or even the odd remark of "you looked better before" do not upset me in the slightest, because I know I am not defined by these negative, rude, or offensive opinions. At first it was hurtful, but I overcame it once my mindset shifted away from allowing myself to be affected by other's opinions of me. I know many people miss out on certain things because they are embarrassed by their body. My fears are now rooted in missing out. I don't want to feel left out for fear of being inadequate. I don't want my shyness or fears of embarrassment to keep me from achieving the things I want to in my fitness journey. Mostly, I don't want to miss out on opportunities to be my true self. I am happiest in an atmosphere where judgment is not present, where everyone can be themselves without hesitation.

The fear of being ridiculed for our bodies or who we are can plague us and leave a permanent wound on our hearts. Often, that wound is self-inflicted. Most of the fears and worries that have held me back are the result of unrealistic expectations. Mostly this comes down to self-doubt and fear of the unknown. The best tack to take is action and effort towards seeking the rewards of self-improvement, whatever they may be. In time, wounds can heal, but for me currently, I am less concerned about healing the wound than with the lasting scars I have made on my heart.

My fears are mostly embedded in a sense of inadequacy. What I have realized is it is not acknowledgement from others I am seeking. It is recognition within myself. For some, I will never be "enough", and that is fine, because the confidence and beauty that comes with being enough for yourself is far more important than anyone else's opinion. There is strength in realizing, knowing, and appreciating your worth and not letting the disparagement of others touch your sense of self. My strength comes from self-acceptance. I remind myself that my body performs with incredible strength day in and day out. I have realized that not looking like the societal standards of beauty does not matter. My body is what it is today and I am who I am today. Today I am enough as is, and so are you.

Facing Your Fears Bucket List

Many of us have "bucket lists" of what we want to do in life, but I don't know anyone with lists of things they never want to do. Many adventure seekers list travel locations, and thrill chasers' lists include bungee jumping or skydiving as bucket list items. I urge you to look at this a different way; I suggest your challenges are personal goals around being positive. For me, it might be wearing shorts confidently on a hot summer day, or carrying on a conversation with a stranger in public. However, it must feel right. This does not mean it will be without hesitation or nerves; you'll know when you are ready. The other day I had a moment to be brave and talk to a stranger, but my heart was racing too fast. I knew my voice would be shaky, so I knew it wasn't time yet. This simply means it was not the right moment for facing that fear. Shyness prevailed that time, but next time can and will be different. I just have to let my truest self shine and realize that growth does not come without discomfort and feeling embarrassed at times.

It is funny to me how much I hate feeling embarrassed, yet I can very easily laugh at myself. Facing fears is scary because there is always that potential of embarrassment, at least for me, but I try to face them to prove to myself how strong and capable I really am. For this exercise, I would like you to make a bucket list of fears that hold you back from reaching your fullest potential. Ask yourself the following questions and set an action plan on how to tackle these current fears. I would love us to celebrate our fearlessness together and encourage you to share your response on Instagram or Twitter. Please use the hashtag #fearlesslymechallenge.

- ° What are things that make you feel vulnerable or exposed to criticism not just from others but from yourself as well?

- ° What makes you shut down mentally and emotionally?

- ° What keeps you from truly being yourself in awkward or embarrassing situations?

- ° What worries or troubles you about your personality? Are you anxious about how you are perceived by others?

- ° How can you learn to embrace these fears in ways that do not let the fear define you?

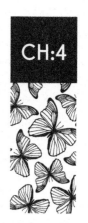

CH:4

More Than a Number

Having embraced a body positive mindset, it is interesting looking back and seeing that at as early as seven years old, I had learned to associate my worth with my appearance and physical capabilities. I was a gymnast for about seven years. Although it was prior to the age when girls tend to become more competitive and catty about appearances, somehow I never felt like I would be good enough for my coaches - I was not the skinniest girl; I was a bit too tall for a gymnast. I was not the most graceful or strongest or best competitor. I was never a "favorite", and that crippled my sense of significance as a team member. Gymnastics is very much an individual sport, but personal performance does dictate overall team rankings, so individuals needed to excel for the team. If you did not excel individually, the team suffered. There was lots of pressure to be the best, and it all revolved around a number.

When I first fell in love with gymnastics, it was about the fun of the sport. I had very strict Russian coaches throughout my whole gymnastics experience, so their expectations on what I should look like and how good I should be were very high. I remember constantly being told I needed to lose 20 pounds at a very young age, and I think made a deep impression in my mind that I was overweight. Looking through old photos I was far from fat. I was muscular and strong. That is just how my body frame is. Skinny does not really fit me, but I always felt like I had to try to be skinny like the other girls on the team.

I look at children today and see their innocence and carefree nature; this always makes me wonder when they will first learn to be insecure and devalued about body shape and size. I was roughly seven when this happened to me. Having coached seven year-olds on a swim team years later, I realized how sad it is to have such a standard placed on us from a young age. There were kids of all shapes and sizes on the team. I heard comments and remarks about certain kids being "bigger." Instead of commending their efforts to be active, they were sometimes ridiculed for even trying because they were not fit enough. Now that I have a different and healthier state of mind, I wish I could go back and stand up for those kids. Hearing offhanded remarks from others on their appearance stung other kids, possibly for the rest of their lives. I know the effects the opinions of others can have on our own self-esteem because I have struggled with it myself, and I hate that children feel devalued because they are "too big" or "not pretty enough." All kids are beautiful. Children should be less concerned with appearances and more concerned with running freely through an open field or swimming in a creek, being carefree and enjoying their innocence as long as possible. No one should ever be made to feel "fat", especially when that person is a child! But around the age of seven, that was my reality, and the doubt that was instilled about my appearance haunted me for a very long time.

Some people are blessed with the gift of good looks their whole life. Others, like me, go through phases. I have had my fair share of awkward and cute phases. I was really awkward and a little chunky when I started gymnastics around age six, but that did not limit my ability. I could still do cartwheels and splits and everything else the other girls on my level could do. From age eight to ten, I had grown and thinned out. I was a little skinny, even. I am sure my confidence and talents grew during this time. But I was not reaching my fullest potential; since I was an obviously fearful child, I was not being pushed in the proper ways. At around eleven, I switched gyms to go to what was considered "the best" gym in my area. Many of the girls I grew up with in gymnastics had switched over to this gym, my best friend included.

It was a tough transition. Many of the girls were in very high levels, some were even elite, and I was only at level five (there are ten levels in gymnasts, six through ten are "open" levels before you become elite). I was older and taller than most of the girls at my level which made me feel uncomfortable. Several of the girls I had started out with in gymnastics quickly leveled up at this new gym, yet I was not really progressing. I needed the challenge, but with challenge came a bit of defeat. Favoritism was strong at this gym, but because I was timid, fearful, and behind on skills, I was rarely a favorite. Nevertheless, the grueling workouts and long gym sessions made me stronger. I learned what it truly took for proper technique. Discipline was elevated here. If I fell off a beam or didn't perform something properly, conditioning consequences would be given. I remember one punishment was to climb a rope, something I never accomplished in all my years as a gymnast. I always felt so defeated because I was too afraid to truly try to master the rope climb. I would exercise for three to four hours a session for three to five times a week, spending roughly thirty minutes to an hour on each event. Every gym session would end with lots of conditioning.

I was definitely in shape during this time. Maybe I was not thin to my coaches' standards, but I was fit, as evidenced by old photos. What my body could do and its flexibility was something I took for granted, because I was too consumed with not being thin enough or strong enough. I didn't see the value in what I could do. I saw my shortcomings for the things I could not do. I remember one time we were practicing front handsprings, a skill set with which I was doing rather well. One of the coaches took note and wanted the other girls to watch me. We were preparing for a state meet competition, so the fact that I was being recognized for something at which I was excelling was thrilling to me.

Before meets, the head coach would watch our performance and give us a score. My mom would often watch in the stands. We reflect back on gymnastics days on occasion, and she told me that the coach would rarely watch me and would throw out some arbitrary number that did not seem to reflect my performance. In the level of gymnastics I was competing in, a 10.0 is a perfect score. So anything in the 9.0+ range was considered excellent. My main focus in switching gyms was to get a 9.0+ on an event because at my old gym I remained anywhere from 6.0-8.0 range, which is sub-par. I put great weight on this number describing my value. I was so excited anytime I got in the 8.0 range, but I knew I could be better. When asked to perform my floor routine at a time when I had been doing well on front handsprings, I was excited and ready to give it my all. The head coach was watching and scoring us that day. Well, the pressure was a bit much, and I ended up rolling my ankle during the front handspring itself. I had to crawl off the floor because it was so incredibly painful. I was not given a score because I could not finish the routine. I was devastated.

My ankle bruised rather badly from this accident, but the timing was in my favor; it happened right before Thanksgiving, so I had a few days to nurse the ankle during the days when the gym was closed for the holiday. I did not go to the doctor though, so a part of me has always wondered if I actually fractured my ankle. Less than a week later, the Saturday after Thanksgiving, I was back in the gym practicing, even though the swelling and bruising had not yet faded. My coaches expressed concern, but I guess it did not hurt enough to force me to continue resting it. I was determined to become my best and get that 9.0+ level.

Because scoring was so important in gymnastics, those little numbers consumed me. My value and worth as an individual depended so heavily on my performance. As a timid gymnast, I would intentionally fall because I was afraid to give it my all. I would psych myself out and scratch on the vault or not catch the higher bar because I was not confident enough to commit. Any fall, wiggle, or wobble was a deduction from your score. You had to be "perfect" to get a higher score. I remember comparing my score to my best friend. I became envious when she started doing better than me, because better scores were naturally higher praised. My jealousy caused a rift in our friendship. It is so sad that I allowed it to get that way. She was a very dear friend and our friendship faded because I could not be happier for her. I was so consumed with my own performance that I forgot to praise others. Naturally, this ended up depleting any self-confidence I had gained. What was the point of excelling if I did not have friends there to celebrate those successes?

I ended up doing well at state competition that year. I finally got a 9.4 on floor. I was so excited, but I was also intensely exhausted. There were many times when I wanted to give up before that moment. I was ready to quit gymnastics many months earlier. But my mom pushed me and made me commit through the end of that season. I am glad she did, because there would have always been a feeling of dissatisfaction for giving up before realizing that potential; that number would have haunted me forever.

The loss of my best friend over feelings of competitiveness bothers me to this day. It was a learning experience; I now see how numbers consumed the majority of my life. I put a heavy weight on numbers and associated those numbers with my significance as an individual. This was my attempt at perfectionism. Sure, getting straight As and succeeding in gymnastics was important to me, but, in the process, I became nothing more than the number I was striving for. I was not good enough if I did not get a 90 or above on an exam or project. I was not good enough if I did not get at least an 8.5 or higher on an event in gymnastics. During my fitness journey,

I came to understand how the idea of numbers defining my worth came from my time as a gymnast.

There is this constant body analysis as a gymnast. Are your muscles flexed enough, butt squeezed tight enough, toes pointed enough? Toes would be slapped if they were not pointed and butts would be poked if they were not clenched. There was continuous pressure to always have our bodies looking a certain way. While watching the women's Rio Olympic trials for gymnastics, it brought back so many positive feelings. Although lots of negativity stemmed from judgment in my childhood, it made me realize several positive things. The bodies of Olympic gymnasts vary greatly. Some are thinner by nature, yet others are powerfully muscular and built, yet both variations are beautiful in their own ways. The power and grace they exhibit is to be admired. Regardless of their build though, I have so much respect for what these women do. Although I was nowhere near their level, having been a gymnast, I know the dedication and personal commitment it requires to be the incredible athletes they are. I have so much admiration and respect for what they can do, and it finally made me realize that my thicker thighs and bigger butt are a gift from my gymnastics days. I am still flexible and still have hidden strength and talent because of all the struggles I went through as a gymnast. I now have a greater respect for my "thicker" build. I have never appreciated having an athletic body more than I have after watching the Olympic gymnasts. It gave me a needed perspective that my body is strong and a reflection of the days when my body did amazing things.

Watching Olympic gymnastics trials has honestly altered my whole viewpoint on my fitness goals. It made me nostalgic for my youth and the abilities I had. I realized that I have been holding myself back because of fear of trying new things. I do not want to be that fearful little girl anymore. Despite the tough realities of an apprehensive youth, I am so thankful I was a gymnast. It gave me the muscular frame I have today. It gave me the strength and flexibility I am still capable of today. It gave me a sense of discipline and ambition for myself. I might not be skinny but my body is capable of doing some pretty hard things. I may still have "problem areas", but they are not limiting me from reaching a more complete fitness potential. Only the mind limits us. It is the fixation and obsession with being a "number" that limits us.

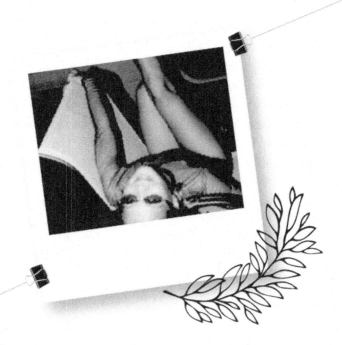

Here is an old image to use as a reference for the days when I was criticized for being "too big" or "needing to lose 20 pounds". I think I was about 9 or 10 here. Looking back on this time, I was in the best shape of my life and certainly do not think I was too big. I think I look fit and strong.

30 Days – No Numbers

A lot of my negative self-talk today stems from the fact that it took me 26 years to separate my worth from my body. I think of all the "would haves," "what ifs," and "could haves," had I been more confident in who I was. I now see I allowed my negative body image to dictate my worth. I put far too much emphasis on the size of my pants, my waist, or even my thighs, and never weighed the value in my personality, traits, or being. I did not weigh or measure the size of my heart. I had always had a strong sense of who I was, but I felt restricted, confined and trapped in a body that did not allow me to fully be me. I allowed that fear factor and shame to consume and control my life.

My whole experience and journey to body positivity has been tied to one thing: worth. I truly believe anyone suffering with self-esteem issues or negative body image is having a difficult time differentiating their worth in who they are from what their body looks like. But I get it! It is very difficult to do. I was there for so long.

I could tell my body was changing roughly eight weeks into my journey. In the beginning, I was obsessed with the scale and watching that number. Once again, I was allowing numbers to define my worth and success. I consistently and healthily lost about a pound a week. But somewhere around week 16, the weight stopped falling off. For MONTHS, that number remained the same and I began to feel defeated. I know I am not alone in this struggle. I follow many young women on similar journeys to my own and am part of Facebook groups dedicated to fitness lifestyles. I see women and girls constantly obsessing over calories and weighing themselves weekly or even daily, and the number never changes or only goes up. The way they react to that is upsetting. I just want to scream, "STOP DEFINING YOURSELF WITH THAT SILLY LITTLE NUMBER!! Stop being so harsh and critical of yourself because those numbers are not changing the way that you wish they would. You are not a number. You are a human with a mind, heart, and soul, and that is what is important, not that number on the scale!" Don't get me wrong, there is merit to paying attention to calories if you want to make effective and lasting changes, but when it becomes an obsession, I feel that is when problems begin. I occasionally still weigh myself but I use it more as a data point and unit of measurement, NOT a unit to define my success or worthiness of existence. I still get frustrated not seeing the scale move because I do work hard trying to improve my body. Why am I putting so much effort into changing myself yet change is not visually happening? I have learned something very important – even though the scale has not changed much in months, change is still happening! My weight and body may not be changing as drastically as in the beginning, but I am getting stronger, my endurance is improving; I am challenging myself in new ways. Maybe my weight is not changing but my heart and mind are. I see a little bit of my younger self in me. One who used to be defined by a number, yet was determined to succeed. I stopped watching the scale and started focusing more on challenging myself to be like a gymnast again, with discipline and determination to become the best version of me. This time would be different. Never again would I define my worth by a number.

I began to focus on having an athletic mindset. I knew I could be better. I could get stronger. I could grow my muscles and become more defined. I wanted to be fit and strong after all! Skinny has never been my goal. After watching the Olympics, I saw the incredible beauty of what it means to be an athlete. I saw the kindness and compassion the athletes had for one another even when one failed to make the Olympic team. The fact that heart prevailed despite failure speaks volumes to what it means to be an athlete. It has nothing to do with looking a certain way, but everything to do with heart, power, determination, and the dedication it takes to be not just an athlete, but a good human being. Most importantly, I have begun to see the beauty I had as a young girl. I see the muscles I possessed as symbol of energy and passion. I am able to see with compassion how my emotions and mind dictated my treatment of others. In this realization, I see how I can now change my mindset and how I value myself. My best self comes from relinquishing the notion of numbers defining my being and treating others the way I want to be treated: with kindness, compassion, respect and care.

Numbers are simply a unit of measurement. But they should not measure your value, worth, or level of attractiveness. We should stop fixing our minds on losing weight simply to see that number decrease and instead focus on figuring out what lies underneath. I have realized this journey was never about losing weight. It has been about dropping insecurities, negative self-talk, fears, hesitations, and reservations. What lies beneath is your truest, most authentic self. It is about clearing your mind of what society says your body should look like and finding out who YOU want to be.

The only numbers that should matter are the amount of your determination, commitment, passion, kindness, and heart for a better you. I think what helped me recover from allowing numbers to consume me was striving to make my inner being more complete and focusing on feeling better about myself. Scales often have a very negative connotation. For this project I would LOVE for you to just dump the scale, but I know for many there is an attachment to checking in and knowing weight as a measurement of progress. I want you to weigh and measure yourself in new ways for this challenge. If you cannot bring yourself to dump the scale, then at least hide it or remove the battery for 30 days. Or place a sticky note over the screen with a note of positivity about how you want to feel after these 30 days. For the next 30 days, focus on these reminders, they can be in any order you choose:

1. Pay yourself a compliment that has nothing to do with appearance.

2. Focus on ways you can gain perspective on how to cultivate an open heart.

3. Give a compliment to a stranger.

4. Determine what a balanced lifestyle means for you.

5. Set a strength goal you want to accomplish.

6. How are you making yourself a priority today?

7. Name something that is difficult for you. Now tell yourself you CAN do it.

8. Ask yourself what feeling you want to accomplish most from living a healthy lifestyle and set realistic steps to move towards that feeling.

9. Set a goal that is not related to physical body improvement.

10. Find a new way to challenge your mind.

11. Get out and tune in with nature; find what sets your soul on fire.

12. Do something that makes you feel vulnerable.

13. Treasure bravery today.

14. Give gratitude for what your body allowed you to do today.

15. Tell someone how you appreciate them.

16. Name a personality trait that makes you authentically you. Try to capture a moment when you are manifesting this trait.

17. Take a moment to choose kindness towards yourself and someone else.

18. Create a mindful motivation that is of a positive influence.

19. Admire someone for their efforts and compliment them.

20. Define what it means to live a happy and healthy lifestyle for YOU and set goals in ways you can reach those goals.

21. What does it mean to be an athlete or champion in your eyes? Is this something you desire to strive for?

22. Set goals to compete with yourself.

23. What things are happening in your life currently that you are thankful for?

24. "It is not what you say, it is how you say it" is a mantra my parents embedded in me. Find ways to speak tenderly to yourself.

25. Define the things you love about yourself that are not appearance related.

26. Step out of your comfort zone today and be sure to give yourself a high five for doing so!

27. What makes your soul FULL?

28. Channel your energies in designing your thoughts in defining your WHO.

29. Focus not on ways to lose weight but on how to tap into your truest self and what makes you uniquely you. Choose individuality!

30. List ways you want to treat yourself with kindness moving forward, and put that list in a place where you can be reminded every day.

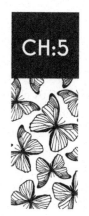

CH:5

Break a Leg

As they were for many people, middle and high school were tough for me. It may seem strange, but I also had a fear of eating in front of others. My theory is that it stemmed from the fear of potentially having to eat alone in the school cafeteria. Many times I would go eat in a favorite teacher's room to avoid eating in the cafeteria during high school. When parties were thrown in class, I would often opt out of eating any treats. Most saw it as remarkable willpower, but looking back, I see it as immense shame and insecurity. I was not particularity bullied or disliked. For the most part, mild cattiness and drama aside, people were kind to me, or nice to my face, at least. However, I held myself back because of the constant negative thoughts in my mind constraining me. I thought it was easier to be unseen than seen. I chose to be invisible. The fear of being judged and disliked by my peers controlled my every move, and it became crippling.

Even though I was uncomfortably shy, I tried to break out of my comfort zone by being a cheerleader from eighth grade through my senior year of high school. I had been a gymnast since I was about 6 to 12 years old. In the previous chapter, "More Than a Number," I talk in more detail about my gymnastics career. I had reached my peak in about seventh grade and was ready to retire as a gymnast. I had had my fill of the sport. I was never going to qualify for a college team, and I was too fearful to try the new skills I was about to learn. I knew it was my time to quit after I finally got the 9.4 on a floor routine at my final state meet. My biggest goal as a gymnast was to score a 9.0+ on an event, and once I achieved that goal, I felt confident enough to leave the sport without regrets. I thought cheerleading was the next best option that would allow me to maintain my flexibility and tumbling abilities, because I was not quite ready to give up all of the skills I had spent the past several years building. However, I now believe that becoming a cheerleader caused me to withdraw more into my insecurities. I was not the skinniest nor the prettiest. I had terrible *bacne* that I was incredibly self-conscious about, and our uniforms often exposed it. As I approached my senior year of high school, my insecurities had taken full control.

I had been seeing a therapist at the time, working through some family issues. I decided to open up to him about the insecurities I had with my body image and how I was afraid to go to college where I felt I was destined to gain the "freshman 15." He referred me to another therapist who dealt with self-esteem, body image, and eating disorders. I saw her up until I began going to college. Ultimately, family problems got worse, and I never attacked the issues behind my negative body image because every session revolved around something else.

Once I settled into my dorm and became familiar with the campus and my classes, I decided I was in control and I had the opportunity to create a new me. I tried to seem outgoing, but my introverted tendencies made it hard to express. I told myself, "This is my chance to truly be me." Unfortunately, it didn't work out that way.

Mine was not the typical college experience. My freshman year was really tough for me, which I believe set the precedent for the remainder of my years in college. I didn't party or go out with the underage drinkers. My family life was at a peak of turmoil, and I was having roommate trouble with my best friend at the time. I just didn't feel comfortable in the dorm, nor did I feel comfortable at home. Mostly I did not feel comfortable with myself. My body, mind, heart, and soul had detached from one another and I was left feeling incomplete. I was deeply worried about my little sister who was drowning in the toxicity of family problems. I wanted to step in and be the support she needed, but it was nearly impossible to pull off while away at college. I often went home on weekends despite how awful it felt just so I could be with my younger sister. At times, we felt like we only truly had each other. When I wasn't worrying about her, I became absorbed in my classes and wanted to excel in school because that was what I thought my family needed.

That was when I began to feed my emotions. I tried to eat well, but since I was on the meal plan, I had access to infinite amounts of treats and comfort foods. When I lived off campus and was not on the meal plan, I resorted to the convenience of fast food and processed foods as meals. At the time, I had little interest in exercising. I would take a class here and there, but used the excuse "I am too busy" to keep myself from establishing some sort of routine. I became my own lowest priority, and for three years I maintained this habit. At that time I also got a part time job as a bus driver, (yes, you read that right, and it was an amazing job,) which began to take away any free time I had to either cook or exercise. Any free time I had was spent on school work. So many evenings I would grab fast food for dinner because of convenience and ease. The weight crept on and the insecurities continued to grow.

I was in complete denial about my weight gain and I avoided scales and mirrors altogether. For the longest time, I would not look at any part of my body except my face in a mirror. I would intentionally dodge them in stores. I avoided full body mirrors like the plague and relied on smaller mirrors to do my makeup in the mornings. My fear of being seen had reached an extreme when I arrived at the point of not even wanting to see myself.

Things did slowly improve though. I was required to take a physical education class as an elective one semester. Since I was in a five-year program, I was advised to wait until my fourth year to take this class due to credit requirements. I reluctantly chose weight training as my P.E. class. It ended up being the one class that fit my schedule best that semester. I thought, "What is the harm in trying something new?" I had about an hour between my classes, so I would often go straight to the gym and do about 40 minutes of cardio before weight training. Twice a week that semester, I did cardio and weights for a total of about a 90 minute workout session.

It took a few weeks, but I started to feel really good. Slowly, I started going to the gym more than twice a week and adding in additional training sessions. I started eating better and feeling better. Unsurprisingly, my family life improved as well. Things were looking up. I still avoided mirrors at all costs, but I was slimming down. By the time finals rolled around, the scales showed I had lost 20 pounds in one semester.

My friends noticed, my family noticed, and most importantly, I noticed, and I was more determined than ever to keep going strong.

During a break between finals, I drove home for a few days to support my little sister's year-end art show. I wanted to get in a workout before the show. Up to this point, all my running and cardio had been on a treadmill. I was excited to finally get outside and enjoy the fresh air on a local greenway I loved. I was ready to really unplug that day and spend some quality time on my own in the great outdoors; I didn't even take my phone on the run. Running outside was a little more difficult than I expected, but I had set a goal to run five miles that day. At the halfway point, I turned to go back and my legs ached. I was tired and had begun shuffling my feet but was determined to not just walk back. The mix of concrete and boardwalks made this greenway tricky with many tripping hazards. On one of the boardwalk sections, I tripped and went down hard. As I fell to the ground, a cracking sound echoed in my ears and the pain instantly flooded my leg. At first I was confused; slowly regaining my composure, I stood back up. I tried walking but couldn't bear any weight on my left leg. Panic immediately set in. I was alone on this run with no one in sight; I didn't even have my phone to call for help.

Fortunately, I was on a popular part of the greenway; I sat and waited for someone to come my way.

A pair of male bicyclists were the first to approach me. They said they did not have their phones on them and that they would bike home and get their wives. They left me there in the hot sun, sweaty, crying, panicky, in pain, and without water. I sat there for another 15 minutes trying to figure out what to do when the next set of people came my way. It was a kindly brother and sister out for a jog. Luckily they had a phone. First, I called my mom. She was out exercising on her lunch break and didn't answer. I tried calling both my dads; neither answered.

A few more people had gathered around and one guy went running towards the fire department, half a mile up the road. The fire department called an ambulance to take me to the hospital, but I refused. I just wanted to get back to my car so I could call my mom on my own phone and go home. I was several yards away from the main road where the fire truck and ambulance had to park. My immediate fear as the firemen approached was, "Oh gosh, they are not going to be able to pick me up." But they did manage, and while being strapped to a gurney, I finally reached my mom. It took a lot of convincing, but I got the firemen to take me to my car. They wanted me to go straight to the hospital in the ambulance but I was insistent. They drove me to my car in the fire truck and gently helped me get into my car.

Once home, I sat in my car until my mom got home. We went straight to the hospital where they took x-rays. There were no signs of a break so the doctors theorized I had possibly torn my ACL or meniscus. An MRI the next day picked up the hairline fracture in my tibia. I was advised to remain off my leg for six weeks until it properly healed.

I received clearance in six weeks to return to normal use of my leg, but my mind decided I wasn't healed nor ready to run again. My leg still did not feel quite right, so I continued to take it easy on my leg. I did not run again or even work out for three years after that.

Naturally, I gained the weight back and lost touch with a regular workout and healthy eating routine. It was not until I started my fitness journey in June of 2015 that I set this fear aside. Risk of injury is still there in the back of my mind at times. But I also know I am mentally strong enough not to let anything hold me back anymore. I used to worry that I would work my ass off for months and get to where I thought I wanted to be only to find my results were not enough. The pain, hurt, and risk of continuing to live in a body you are unhappy with far exceeds any fear of discontentment you might find "at the end." The process of learning to know yourself and love yourself makes any struggle incredibly worthwhile.

I look at old pictures of myself from my time in college; I can now see I didn't look as bad as I thought. I probably weighed 20 pounds less than I do now, yet the unhappiness in my face is so apparent. I see now silly it was to let such angst about my body take precedence above all else. Yes, I still have insecurities and things I wish to change, but now I simply acknowledge them and am content in knowing that I am still working towards being my best. It is so easy to get caught up in the "what ifs" or "should have/would haves" of a fitness lifestyle and routine. There are so many times I could have worked out harder or eaten better. I choose not to dwell on that, because the simple fact is that every day I wake up and make health and happiness a priority by doing my best each day. I look back on my high school days and simply laugh at how embarrassingly shy I was over the littlest of things. I am thankful for all that has happened to me. It made me the strong, independent, tough-willed and determined person I am today.

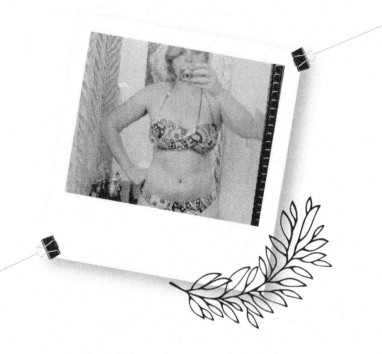

This is a photo I took as a "before" pic right before I tried doing the program insanity. Looking back, the only thing I see wrong with this image is the sadness and dissatisfaction in my face. This is a good reminder of how time, growth, perspective, and a little self-love can change how we view ourselves. One thing to remember is that body dissatisfaction does not discriminate on body shape or size. It can happen to anyone and you have the power to do something about it.

Create a Setback Plan

Things rarely go exactly as planned. You could have
your week or day planned out to a T, but all it takes is the
slightest change and your daily or weekly efforts seem
to be completely derailed. We get sick. We get injured.
Unexpected things occur. We get busy. We get run down.
We get comfortable. The key to making lasting and effective
change is one thing: consistency. A day, a weekend, or
even a week off track is nothing in the grand scheme of
life. After a day or two, it is easy enough to simply get back
on track with a regular routine. Six weeks to heal from a
major injury requires time to get your groove back. For this
challenge, I want you to create a setback plan. This will
serve as an excellent reminder for when you deviate from
your routine for longer due to injury, illness, or life taking
an unexpected turn. Maybe you are really busy with travel,
or it's finals week, and eating right and exercising is the
last thing on your mind. That is OK! Because life happens.
Just don't let it become an ongoing excuse, because that
is when old habits resurface and become constant. My
question to you is this: if the unexpected happens, what
steps will you take to get back into your routine? I suggest
you start slowly and gradually build back to where you
were. If you try to tackle too much at once, it can become
overwhelming. Remember to be patient, gentle, and kind
with yourself while you begin to get back into your healthy
routine. It might require establishing healthy habits again;
just remember it is just as easy to form good habits as it is
to form bad habits. The choice is yours in how you choose
to overcome those unexpected moments. You can let this

define and consume you, or you can rise and become your own phoenix by being better than your excuses. Just don't do what I did and wait three years to get back into a healthy routine. Have a game plan ready today so that you are prepared for the unexpected.

CH:6

Your Best

I remember the very moment when I truly understood the meaning of my step-dad's words. He would always tell me, "Swimming is 10 percent physical, and 90 percent mental." I had just finished a 50 yard freestyle swim. I was completely exhausted, yet I felt great because I had just pushed myself like I never had before. As I began to regain awareness of my surroundings after catching my breath for a few seconds, I slowly pulled myself out of the pool. I could hear my step-dad yelling, "GREAT SWIM, JESS! GREAT SWIM!" I looked over and saw his excitement, so I ran over to see what he had clocked for my time. It was roughly 30.4 seconds! In that moment, I knew exactly what it felt like to be my very best.

Now, 30.4 seconds for a 50 yard freestyle swim is not even close to an Olympic qualification time, but it was so close to my personal goal of swimming this event in under 30 seconds. We were at one of my preferred meets at one of my favorite pools, the Green Street pool in Gainesville,

Georgia. I loved meets there because they were bigger, with amazing swimmers attending from all over north Georgia. The competitive edge at these meets inspired me to push myself. Freestyle and butterfly were my best strokes; I would use these to really try for my best time at Green Street meets. Anxiety brought on nausea, self-doubt and constantly rechecking my event, heat, and lane numbers to make sure I showed up in time. My mom did her best to ease my nerves and remind me, "It's just a race." She was so right. This pool had electronic timing water pads, and our times would be accurately clocked and printed out on a board. Excitedly, I would look to see if I had knocked any time off my time last years. Even if it was .02 seconds, it was a win to me. I always felt like I had to prove something to myself. Once again, a number measured my worth.

This round, I was extra nervous. My heart was racing, my hands and feet were sweaty, my mouth was dry. But I was ready. I remember cautiously stepping up onto the dive block. I made a point to remind myself to relax and take a deep breath while waiting for the cue to take my mark. Before I knew it, I was in diving position. The beep sounded and I leaped off into the frigid water. I kept telling myself, "It's only 30 seconds. It's only 30 seconds. You don't need to breathe. Fight the pain. Fight the exhaustion. You can take a few more strokes without a breath." It may sound odd, but fewer breaths does help contribute to a faster time because of a more streamlined swim. I had been training to time my breath and condition my lungs. My step-dad had always told me to never take a breath the first stroke off the turn, and I tried it during this race. I waited three to five strokes before taking a breath. I could feel it; I just knew that all the training had led up to this moment, and it worked for me beautifully. From that moment on, I no longer needed to compete with anyone else. I no longer wanted to be faster than the other girls, I simply wanted to be faster than my previous self.

From grade school through high school, I swam on the neighborhood swim team that my step-dad coached for many years. I swam only during the summer, which meant that every summer I had to get back to where I was the previous summer and then go from there. I remember one summer really wanting to excel. At the pool, my step-dad was the coach, and I respected him as such. I told him I wanted to get my best times and beat my times from the last year. As a coach, he would often split up the lanes based on ability and push the swimmers in each lane in the ways that were best for them. This particular summer, I was pushed exceptionally hard. During a timed interval session, I became really frustrated because I could not hit the intervals. We were doing 50 yard freestyle sprints on the 45 seconds, which meant that if it took 40 seconds to sprint the 50 yards, then we would only get a 5 second rest. These intervals encouraged you to swim faster to get a little longer break, even if you were more winded by the extra effort. On this particular day, I was really struggling. The stress of it started getting me down and I began to cry. Coach was not sympathetic. He told me, "You want to be your best? You want to beat your times from last year? Suck it up and push through. Even if you do not get any rest, just keep sprinting." In that moment I disliked him, but I also knew he was right. I could have easily gone home and sulked, but I pushed through and finished that intense sprint set. These moments of mental and physical breakthrough are necessary for my personal growth. As much as it sucked in the moment, it made me a better, stronger, and faster swimmer that year. It helped me become my best that season.

Out of all the sports I have participated in, swimming was hands down my favorite. Once in a while I wonder to myself, "What if I had quit cheerleading and focused more on swimming? How different would things be today?" I didn't swim year-round because the only indoor practice pool was 45 minutes away, which required early mornings and late nights. Sideline cheerleading was very social; it was all about spirit fingers, excitement, and wondering who stole whose pompoms. Swimming was simply you becoming one with the water. The only time I really remember feeling any insecurity as a swimmer was my last summer before college. My best friend was swimming and coaching as well. We set a goal to lose some weight before heading off to college. She succeeded in losing 15 pounds. I lost none. I found myself comparing myself to her; why couldn't I do it?

Thinking back on my sports days, I always had coaches telling me what to do, how to exercise and pushing me to become my best. When I left for college, I didn't have anyone encouraging me. I was on my own. I thought weight loss and getting into shape was all about motivation. What I now know is that it takes willpower and the desire to change. Changing your lifestyle is less about motivation and more about self-control. As a swimmer or gymnast, I was coached and conditioned to be disciplined in my practice. There were days when I felt so weak, I was sure I could not complete the practice. Even in those times, I still pushed through and did the best I could in the moment. The excuse

I gave myself as to why I could not lose weight was that I was not changing my eating habits. For me, changing eating habits comes from an understanding of how to eat properly and desire to be healthier, not skinnier.

As I reflect on this journey, I understand that I lacked structure, organization, and knowledge of how to take care of myself on my own. I didn't have someone telling me what to do or how to do it. I did not have workouts magically written out for me to follow. For many years, I floundered around trying to "figure healthy out." How many of us can afford a personal trainer? Not many. And training with a sports coach is still very different than with a trainer, because the exercises and results are very different. Weight training is often about sculpting your body to look a certain way, while swimming on the other hand is more about conditioning your body to work more in a more streamlined and efficient way in the water to achieve a faster time. Because I took weight training in college, I know my way around the weight room. But when it comes to creating an actual workout that is efficient? I. Am. Clueless.

I think many people are fearful about the first time at a gym because of the lack of experience factor, or worse yet, the possibility of looking ridiculous. The truth is, we ALL start somewhere. I started out following a 12-week guide that helped me keep on for over 60 weeks consistently. The plan worked well for me because it was very organized and structured; the guidelines told me what to do. I didn't have my step-dad, a coach, or a trainer keeping me accountable, I only had myself. It can be daunting getting into shape. It can be so difficult. It can be overwhelming. But it is possible. It can be accomplished. It CAN be done, by you.

On days when I am lacking motivation, it is really energy and inspiration I need. For me, loss of motivation is more of a boredom with the routine. If something is no longer fun or challenging, then it is time to switch things up or challenge yourself in a new way. I feel this way a lot, so I have to constantly mix it up. I look for inspiration online. Most of my current inspiration actually comes from male athletes. It might seem a bit odd, but I am constantly amazed by what I see some of the guys are capable of doing. From them, I have learned not to say, "I wish I could do that," or "I can never imagine doing that," or "Never in my wildest dreams would I accomplish something like that." Instead I say, "How can I learn and challenge myself to do *that*!?" or "I really want to do one armed pushups and handstand pushups. How do I get there? I know I can!" This is how I challenge myself now. It is so important to a healthy lifestyle to never stop challenging yourself and always remain a student. Strive to learn what you are capable of.

Often people think they need a trainer to reach their fitness goals. While working with a trainer has many positive merits, it is not always practical. Some people are busy with jobs, families and travel commitments; others can't afford a monthly gym membership. It doesn't have to cost a lot of money to get into shape, but it does at times require some creativity. If you don't have a trainer showing you the ropes around the gym, supporting you, and cheering you on, how do you succeed? Even if you have no basic knowledge of exercise, you can get started by doing some research. There are so many easy programs and tools online that it may take some effort to find the one that best suits your needs. Find one that looks like it will fit your schedule and your goals and also is within your ability range. Compare user reviews of programs that interested you. Reach out to people asking for honest advice and feedback on the program you are considering. Remember to always follow the requirements set out in the guide. If you are unsure how to do something, just ASK someone. If you are working out at home, research how to do it properly. When you don't have a coach perfecting form or movements, it can be easy to do something incorrectly and injure yourself. It is very important to make sure you follow the instructions in whatever guide or program you choose to follow and that you are doing it safely. Most importantly, be realistic in your goals and work from your current capabilities. Do not commit to some insanely difficult program if you have never worked out before in your life. Even if you do not want to follow a strict program because you feel "too out of shape," go for a 30 minute walk or find a group exercise class a few days a week. Just move your body in the best way you can today. The opportunities are endless.

What you eat is also key when it comes to changing your lifestyle, and this is often the trickiest part. I don't have a background in nutrition and admit to binging episodes, but I always knew that a combination of eating right and exercising would help me accomplish my initial goal to be healthier. Nutrition can be so confusing, but don't let yourself be overwhelmed. Start by changing one small unhealthy habit a day. It can be anything. For some example, if you drink soda, try giving up soda for the day, or having one less soda a day. Instead of getting a whole milk full fat latte and donut from your local coffee shop, opt for a skim milk latte and oatmeal. Before heading to the office, pack a lunch four days a week instead of eating out every single day. It really is the little things. Repeat this. Every. Single. Day. Suddenly all these little changes add up and amount to a bigger transformation. By changing one small thing a day, you will end up with big results over time. In the long run, it is about becoming better as you go. The best thing about living a healthy and active lifestyle is that you are allowed to change routines and try new things along the way. Your evolution and transformation would be far less meaningful if everything happened all at once. The beauty in the journey is witnessing your change in not just the physical aspect, but in mental and emotional improvements, as well.

In my swimming career, I never swam a 50 yard freestyle in under 30 seconds. This could seem like a failure, but I still see it as an opportunity. Sure, I am older now, but age is just a number, not an excuse for not trying. I know what training it takes to get there and what I need to do. In the past, I have made excuses like, "Oh, the gym with the large pool is too far away, and I don't want to go out there just to swim." But here's the thing, I will never swim an under-30-second 50 yard freestyle just by talking about it. It requires doing. It requires action. This takes real effort, consistency, dedication, discipline, moxie, and fortitude to get there. I now have to be my own coach, and my own cheerleader as well. Truth to be told, you have to cheer for yourself, because most of the time no one else will do it for you. Even if you feel like you were defeated in a workout, still commend yourself and your efforts. After all, you gave it your best and got out there and tried.

When I started my journey, I only committed to the initial 12 weeks. I figured it would require much more time than that to get to my ultimate goals, but I saw it as a kickstart to get back into some sort of routine. Most online programs are 90 days, or roughly 12 weeks. Think about how long a lifetime is. 12 weeks in a lifetime is NOTHING. By week 8 into this program. I had fallen in love with the process. It became habit. But it took a lot of energy as well as defeat, soreness, being winded, and feeling so out of shape. I had times when I thought exercise just was not meant for me. On one occasion I was on the floor for most of the workout, but I still gave myself credit because I made myself a priority that day, even though I didn't want to. I carried around a printout of the program that I used; that little piece of paper became my de facto coach. When I started seeing results in week 8, I became my own cheerleader. I learned to support, motivate, and encourage myself during the good times and the bad. Mostly, I cheered for self-love all through the highs and lows of the process.

It took many months for me to realize this was my *own* race. I cannot compare this journey to anyone else's but my own. The most important thing I have learned is how much BEAUTY and POWER comes from owning your individuality and your perfectly placed flaws. Every journey is unique, and it is so important to simply focus on striving to become YOUR best in anything and everything you set out to accomplish.

Mirror Mantra

Create a mirror mantra to recite to yourself either every morning or every night or before a workout, whichever will be more motivating for you. Try a tone or a voice other than your own. Use a past coach, a motivator, a loved one, or someone who inspires you to be the voice of your mantra. It may seem silly to not use your own voice, but I have found we tend to be our own worst detractors and can often be overly self-critical. Using the tone of another's voice can be more gentle, respectful, kind, and encouraging. Consider the qualities your loved ones and friends admire in you and use those in your mantra. Think of the things you also love about yourself that are not physical traits and use them in your mantra as well. Make it loving. Make it positive. Your mantra should embody strength, dignity and grace. Whatever you come up with, make sure it is self-empowering! Write it down and tape it where you will see it every day in the bathroom mirror. You can also write your mantra on post-its, take them to work, and stick them on your monitor or where you see can see them in your work space. Recite these words of self love out loud to yourself until you feel the words to be true and believe them in your heart. Be sure to include this line at the end: "Do not forget to love yourself today. You are worthy and you are enough as you are today and all the days to follow."

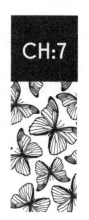

CH:7

Abs or Memories?

"Ladies and gentlemen, this is your captain speaking. We are about 81 miles away from Austin. The control tower is currently being flooded due to inclement weather, so we cannot land and are being rerouted to San Antonio. Flight attendants, prepare for landing." As a person who suffers from generalized anxiety, the next 20 or so minutes were agonizing. Panic quickly set in and negative thoughts flooded my mind: "Where is San Antonio in relation to Austin? Can I drive? Will it be safe to drive? Am I going to be stranded here? Will tomorrow be wasted traveling?" I was supposed to land in Austin at about 11:25 p.m. to meet some of my Instagram friends for a girls' weekend; I would be meeting two of them for the first time. It was then 1:00 a.m. and we had just landed in San Antonio. Earlier that day, I got up at 4:45 a.m. to get my workout in early and take my dog to a board and care before work that day. I was a bit too exhausted to drive since I had been up so early that morning, but I was determined to stay awake until I made it to Austin.

Seconds after we landed, I called the friend I was staying with. She answered excitedly, "You just landed!" I replied, "Yeah, but unfortunately in San Antonio, not Austin." She exclaimed, "WHAT? The board here says you just landed here." We chatted for about 30 minutes trying to figure out what was going on. She was being told that we were just going to park for a few minutes to let the weather in Austin clear up before we lifted off again for Austin. On my end, we had been sitting on the runway for over an hour waiting for a gate to open up so we could deplane. Once we finally got off the plane, we were not being told anything, but my friend was still being told we were going to take off again in about 30 minutes.

A young woman from my flight had reserved a car while we were sitting on the runway. Another young woman asked what I was doing. I was conflicted. I thought about getting a car, but since I had not reserved one, I was worried that none would be available for me. The girl who had reserved one approached us and said we were welcome to ride with her. I was hesitant because I was hopeful our flight would take off soon. I didn't want to leave without my luggage, and I was not sure if or when it would get there. Finally I decided I didn't want to be stranded in San Antonio and that my luggage would probably arrive sometime the next day.

The woman who had reserved the car called to confirm her reservation, because once we left the airport, we could not get back in with security closed for the night. We were confident we had a car, so we left anyway. Once we arrived at the car rental office, there was only one attendant at the desk helping a customer, with only one more guy in line in front of us. It was nearly 2:30 a.m. A woman came to help out at the desk and assisted the man in front of us who had also been on our flight. Pretty much everyone at the car rental was taking a one-way trip to Austin.

The guy ahead of us at the counter was a bit sketchy and was being difficult. He had no reservation and was requesting a luxury vehicle for a one-way 90 minute trip to Austin. Why he wanted a luxury vehicle for such a short trip at almost three in the morning was mystifying. People in line remarked on how strange it seemed. By this point, the line was also beginning to lengthen considerably. The car rental agent made an announcement: "For those of you who have reserved a vehicle for a one-way trip to Austin in the last four hours, I can no longer guarantee you a vehicle. We have to allow the customers who have made a more advanced reservation priority at this time as we are running out of vehicles."

The other women and I were alarmed. What were we going to do? How were we going to get to Austin? We could not go back to the airport because we could not get back to the gate! The guy renting the luxury vehicle wrapped up his reservation. He gave us a smirk and with a "see ya" gesture, walking toward the door. Then one of the young women in our little group half-jokingly yelled, "If you are going to Austin, can we come with you!" He turned around and said, "Yeah, sure!" At first, we thought he was kidding, but he was actually sincere in his offer. The other women and I looked at one another with both uncertainty and relief as we agreed to go with him.

We got into the car before him, since he had to get the keys. I turned to the other women and anxiously whispered, "I don't have the best vibe from him; do we trust him? What if he is a terrible driver? Or worse, some sort of criminal!" One of the women replied with, "What other choice do we have? It's three of us women against one. I think we are pretty safe. Sure, he seems a bit pompous, but I think he is probably okay." I knew she was right, and I really did not have another option. As exhausted as I was, I made sure I remained awake and alert to whether anything suspicious seemed to be happening.

Once on the road, we all began talking and listening to each other's stories and reasons for going to Austin. Our driver had been traveling from Seattle and landed in Dallas for a connection flight which was also detoured to San Antonio. We found out that he had managed to get a car without a reservation because he had lied to the desk attendant that he was proposing to his girlfriend the next day and really needed to get to Austin. I guess "bro code" really worked to his advantage. He had a 7:00 a.m. meeting to attend, so I sympathized, and his little lie had ultimately helped the other young women and I. I told the group I was traveling to Austin to meet people I had met on Instagram for the first time, which sounded really crazy to them. The other two women were traveling there for a girls' weekend as well.

Nothing too eventful happened on the drive. We arrived in Austin around 4:30 a.m., exactly when our flight arrived from San Antonio, enabling me to pick up my luggage after all. Whether I stayed at the airport or traveled with strangers, I still ended up at my final destination, safe and sound. In the moment, it felt riskier to stay and wait for my flight. I was not confident it was going to leave that night. It was *way* out of my comfort zone to agree to travel with people I didn't know from my flight via car; in retrospect, I came away with a great story and I got a chance to grow that day. The old, insecure shy me would have played it safe and risked not making it to Austin that night. The new me embraced a little adventure and allowed me to step out of my comfort zone in a way I never would have expected.

My sweet pals had stayed at the airport all night waiting for me. One of them had to work half a day that day and was a true champ staying up all night waiting for me. As we were leaving, it was about 5 a.m. Coffee shops were just starting to open and that became our biggest priority. The adventure was still on though. My other friends coming in from California had still not made it yet. They had been directed to Dallas, about three hours away, and were going to rent a car as well. But as luck would have it, they ended up finding an Uber driver willing to take them from Dallas to Austin. These were the women I had yet to meet and I was filled with happy anticipation. I had met the two Texans in December at a New York Instagram get together. They were my surprise roommates then and we have been great friends ever since.

My California friends made it in around 6:30 a.m. Exhaustion was replaced with exuberance as we jumped and hugged and laughed until our friend had to leave for work. While she left, we finally passed out for a nap. It might sound wacky meeting up with total internet strangers like we were best friends who haven't seen each other for a long time, but these connections and friendship are very real and genuine. The vulnerability and truth these women share on their pages makes me realize we are all human. They are honest about who they are, and I was not at all afraid I would be meeting someone different than they presented online.

When I created my fitness account on Instagram, I had one intention only - to be accountable to myself. I had zero expectations of what was to follow. I was afraid to put myself out there and show such unflattering pictures of my body, figuring, "Really, what is the worst that can happen?" I did worry about people I knew finding me and learning of my deep internal struggles with body image and self-esteem. I knew there was the possibility of internet trolls bringing me down. Though both of these things happened, I am stronger because of it; because the more I open up and share my rawest and most vulnerable moments, the more connected I feel. I didn't expect girls and women to reach out to me and say, "I feel this way too!" Knowing I am not alone with my internal battle has made every ounce of discomfort worthwhile.

The best thing that has come out of having an Instagram fitness account was the most unexpected thing I could have ever imagined: friendship. I am not talking acquaintances that I interact with on the internet on occasion. I mean real, genuine, true-life friendships that span the United States and the WORLD. It is mind-boggling how an app led me to find some incredible women who have become some of my closest friends. Before my journey, my roommate was pretty much the only friend I could really rely on in Florida. Since then, I have connected with so many other local women who are willing to meet up for a workout or a healthy brunch, or even to go for a girls' night out of cocktails and dancing. We all share similar vulnerabilities and insecurities, but mostly we share the same passion for living a healthy and active lifestyle. I knew when I met up with these women in Austin that they would be willing to work out or grab a healthy smoothie instead of something less nourishing, because we share a similar lifestyle. I also knew if laziness or pizza was the order of the day, they would be down for that, too. Most importantly, I knew there would be no judgment in any way, shape, or form. And that understanding allowed me to let my soul be completely free that weekend. I had never felt more like myself.

The biggest thing that trip taught turned out to be some of the most important words I have learned during my entire journey: balance and flexibility. Exercise is something I crave and really and truly enjoy. Gym time is my favorite time of the day. I really look forward to it, and some days I count down the hours until I can get my sweat on. I did not start out this way, though. It took many weeks of forcing myself to do so to get into a routine. There were days when I would sit on the gym floor for quite some time waiting for the room to clear out, because I was too embarrassed to work out with people around me. Once I got a good routine going, I became more confident, and my new initiative became a habit. I fell in love with living an active lifestyle, which ultimately helped me learn to love myself in ways I never expected. I did not see exercise as a chore, I began to see it as something my body deserved. Exercising is a way of respecting your body, your whole self. Now, I don't exercise just to change my physical self, I exercise to stay healthy and reward my body for all the things it does for me daily.

In the beginning of my journey, I stopped going out for fear that I would party too hard, then eat late night pizza and lose all my progress in a night of indulgence. Sure enough, I began to feel isolated and lonely again, because I was not enjoying life. I overcorrected and made working out and a food regime too much of a priority. Nourishment also comes in the form of laughter, fun, happiness, and making new memories. Living a healthy lifestyle is not a fad. It is not a diet. It is not temporary. If what you are doing is not sustainable for a long time, you are at risk of old, unhealthy habits resurfacing. Exercise is hard, especially when you are out of shape. I get it, really I do, because I have been there more than once. I am not sure exercise is meant to ever be easy, but it still can be *fun*. It can be very challenging, but use the challenge to test your abilities. There is nothing more empowering than realizing you *can* do something you thought you never could do. It truly is a LIFE style and something that is meant to be maintained for a long period of time. This does not mean what you are doing now is for forever, things can change. This is where balance and flexibility are key so that you can be content with trying new things and figuring out what works better and then best for you.

Prior to this journey, I hated my body. I criticized my thighs for how big they were, how dimply they looked, or how much they jiggled when I walked. I would often pinch my stomach because I wished I could just cut off the fat that I loathed. Worse, I used this as an excuse for why I was unworthy and undeserving of so many different things. There are still times even today when I criticize myself or still wish this or that would change faster. The minute I realize this is happening, I remind myself of this important thing. A balanced and flexible life style is so much more than simply eating right and exercising every day, because although I might not love my legs today, they carry me even when I feel my lowest. Our bodies are simply ephemeral, but our souls are everlasting. I take care of my body because it is home to my soul, and I take care of this home so that my soul can thrive.

Living a healthy and active lifestyle means nothing if you are not working on nourishing your mind, heart, and soul as well. You could have the "prettiest" body, but if your heart and mind do not reflect that inner beauty, what is the point in looking nice? I have found that this fitness journey is not just about transforming my body; it is about a holistic experience of moving towards the best version of me as a complete being both physically and spiritually. Balance is not about being able to do a handstand. Balance, for me, means sustaining my body with healthy foods and exercise as close as possible to 80% of the time, yet feeding my mind and heart with meaning, connection, and conversation. Flexibility is far more than just being bendy and able to do the splits. Flexibility, for me, is allowing the spaces between my mind, heart, and soul to be open to different energies and the fluidity of change.

Balancing Flexibility

There is so much more to life than simply eating kale and greens all the time while exercising an hour every day. Life would be meaningless without memories, and it is important to consider your goals and how much you are sacrificing. It is important to enjoy life and work that into your plans. For many, balance in diet comes from "cheat meals." Personally, I don't like the idea of cheat meals simply because that mindset has you "looking forward" to a certain time or meal. Instead, I prefer to live in the moment. If friends want to go out, I try not to say no and accommodate my schedule accordingly. Sometimes I will opt for a salad and other times I will order the cheesiest slice of pizza. It all depends on my mood and allowing myself to live in the moment without fear of regretting a decision I made about food. Flexibility comes from either thinking ahead or simply reorganizing my week if something comes up out of the blue that I want to participate in. Other times it is learning when to say no and when to say yes. I say yes if I think I will regret not accepting, I say no if I think missing out on an experience will not affect me later. But what works for me in terms of balance and flexibility may not work for you. That is why it is important to establish *your* sense of balance and flexibility and what you think will work best for you.

I think for balance and flexibility to work best, they simply need to become a habit, an established routine. However, I know some people do not thrive on structure, as they prefer a little spontaneity. I view routine as the balance and flexibility as the spontaneous bit. I think you can and should have a little of both. I am a visual person, so I need to see and make a list of what is most important to me; I find it helpful to establish a hierarchy in my daily and weekly routines. For this exercise, simply fold a piece of paper in half and label one side balance and the other side flexibility.

For **balance**, write out the key words that are your non-negotiable items. These are the things that will be routine, things you do daily. Even if you are not all that structured or scheduled, there are some things you have to do. I want YOU to be the first and biggest priority on this balance list.

For **flexibility**, write out the key words that are your negotiable items. These are the things that are the spontaneity bit or the things you enjoy doing. How do they fit in with balance? Where can things begin to move around? Make whatever is most important to you your top priority.

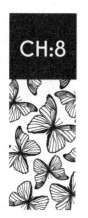

CH:8

Searching for Happiness

The biggest reason why I started my fitness journey was that I wanted to feel happy. I was in a very dark place for a few months leading up to my breaking point. I worked at a job that left me feeling worthless, talentless, unmotivated, lonely, melancholy, and desperate for change. I did not know this change would be through self-discovery; I simply thought the difference would come from changing work environments. I thought changing my body as well as changing jobs would help with feeling happier. I felt insufficient at my job but also with myself. I had forgotten who I was, because I had previously associated so much of my worth with my artistic talents. When those talents came into question, I began to doubt and question myself. After I started my new job, I thought it would be the perfect time to focus on myself and what could make me happier. I knew the change in environment was necessary, but I also thought losing weight would help make me feel better, too. Little did I know that happiness was much deeper than the surface.

During my "quarter life crisis" as I call it, there were many times I intentionally isolated myself. At the time, I really only had one friend I could rely on in Florida. She is my roommate and my best friend. I am not one to break down and cry in front of others, it is too intimate and that makes me uncomfortable. Once, I got home from work and just sat outside in my car and wept. My roommate noticed I had pulled into the driveway and when I didn't come in for a long time, she came out to check on me. She was so patient and gentle during that time period and was the only person to witness the change in me. No one saw me struggle like she did. When she found me crying in my car, she said "I miss you," even though I was right there. I knew exactly what she meant. I missed me too.

My lowest point during this mentally trying time was when my roommate, her boyfriend, and a few other people I knew attended a soccer game without me. I had declined their invitation since I thought I had no interest in soccer, then I instantly regretted not going when I felt left out and lonely. I had no one to blame but myself. I was missing that connection to others and I failed to see how simply allowing myself to be present would have helped with the immense sadness I was feeling at the time. Just before changing jobs, I had biked from my house to the newly opened neighborhood Sunrail station and took the train to my old office. This was a bit adventurous for me, and I felt like I was actually living a more urban experience. It was new. It was different. It was out of my comfort zone. The day everyone was at a soccer game, I biked the mile and a half to the station for the first time. On my way home, I noticed a man walking along the side of the road. I did not really think anything of it until he stopped me. He was

Planking For Pizza

clearly confused and disoriented and this made me a little nervous. He asked to use my phone because his friends had left him alone at a house party the night before in an area he was unfamiliar with. His phone had died. His watch was missing. This was clearly was a "walk of shame." Once I realized he was not going to harm me, I felt sorry for the guy; we all have had those regrettable moments. I let him use my phone to call a friend who never answered. He became a bit flustered, saying he didn't know where he was, how to get home, and needed to get to work in just a few hours.

Because I was feeling particularly lonely that day, I did something very uncharacteristic for me. I was only about a quarter mile from home, so I offered to bike home, grab my car and drive him home. Clearly I was *not* thinking. Once I got home, I was thinking, "This is a terrible idea. Should I take protection? What if he is a bad guy and preying on me because I am being nice? I could just not go back. It's not like he followed me home or would know where I lived. Maybe I should grab my dog Coosa. Surely he would protect me, right?" Coosa in tow, I got in the car and rolled down my window, thinking I would be protected by screaming in case he tried to harm me. This all seemed perfectly logical at the time.

Once I returned, he got in the car he proceeded to explain why he was so disoriented. At the house party, they had downed bottles of whiskey and popped ecstasy pills all night. He didn't remember much of anything about the actual events of the night. I suspected he was still high even though it was about two in the afternoon. I started thinking, "What have I gotten myself into? This is so stupid.

This is how I am going to die, by being nice and picking up a stranger off the side of the road. Cool, Jess, cool." I try to not judge others for the things they do or mistakes they may have made, but here was a stranger who was openly talking to me about doing drugs while I was alone with him, not knowing anything about him.

At last, I got the guy home safely and he thanked me profusely. Even though I was nervous the whole time, I actually felt pretty good because I had done something nice. But I followed it up with something pretty lousy; I lied to my friend, saying I had gone inside with the guy, which was not true at all. I don't entirely understand why I felt the need to lie. I suppose in a way it was a tactic to make me feel of importance and value to my friends who were having fun without me. It was wrong of me to do and definitely my way of having a pity party.

Suddenly, I realized how lonely I truly was. Picking up a stranger off the side of the road? That was desperate. I really was in a low place. I should have started seeking therapy at the time, but it hadn't yet crossed my mind that I needed professional help for the feelings I was having. I am no stranger to therapy, having gone every week from ages five to ten and again in high school. In fact, I truly believe it will always be a part of my life. I learned how to cope with family problems as well as emotional and behavioral issues. Oftentimes in therapy, you are given homework assignments to work on the things you are learning to deal with. In a recent therapy session, I brought up how that all previous sessions had only covered my family problems and how to deal with those feelings. I had never talked about how I felt about myself.

I remember one of my long-term homework assignments as a child was with printouts of thermometers. One was labeled "angry" and the other labeled "sad." I had to color in the angry one with red and the sad one with blue to express just how much I felt either or both emotions. While discussing this with my current therapist, I realized that there was no "happy". My therapist asked, "So, where was the happy? Were you not happy?"

Thinking back, I definitely had happy moments, but I was not the happiest child, and the "angry" and "sad" emotions carried on throughout the years. I began to wonder, had I ever truly known what "happy" feels like? I asked my mom if there had been a happy thermometer, just out of curiosity. She could not remember exactly, but she thought there were "happy" and "neutral" thermometers as well. But she stated that angry and sad were the ones they were mostly concerned with because it was hard to tell how I was actually feeling a lot of the time. Looking at old photos, I rarely look genuinely happy. I remember moments of happiness from my past, but I truly do not think I ever was really happy.

Feeding Anxiety

In high school, I began to experience physical ailments which I now know were manifestations of my anxiety. They began shortly before a big art history trip to Italy. I experienced a great deal of nausea, couldn't eat, and then "nervous tummy" digestion issues followed. I had extreme dry mouth, too. The weirdest sensation of all was a numbness and tingling in my chest. It started happening frequently, and I became scared that I was getting really sick. It began two months before this trip. I thought for sure once I got back it would all ease, but it didn't happen. I went to a general practitioner afterwards to make sure nothing more extreme was happening. She diagnosed me with depression and prescribed an antidepressant. My mom and I disagreed with her diagnosis and refused to fill the prescription. Looking back though, maybe that doctor was right. Maybe I was depressed and was simply unwilling to accept it.

There were so many times when I let anger, frustration, anxiety, or sadness control my actions. I remember one embarrassing moment as a teenager when I really allowed my emotions to take over. My family organized and ran our neighborhood swim; for eleven years, it was a fun summer family bonding experience.

One day at practice I became quite angry. I don't remember exactly what happened, but I know it was during the transition years when my little sister was slowly taking over the 10 and under age group as their head coach. I used to coach that group with when the team was young, and I had formed quite an attachment with them. My step dad told me to relinquish control and allow my sister to lead as coach and I didn't like that one bit. By then, I was a moody teenager, feeling thwarted, but looking back on it,I sense there were deep-rooted feelings involved. I exchanged some very loud and unkind words with my step-dad in public. It was embarrassing for my family and for me, but thankfully we were a small family-run / family-oriented team. After my inexcusable behavior, I ended up storming off, and drove home and locked myself in my room. I ended up in a fetal position on the floor, bawling my eyes out. It sounds dramatic, but looking back, this is how I handled things. I did not know how to control myself or how to respond when my emotions felt out of balance.

I also recall times when anxiety took over and controlled my reactions around food, which always happened around my biological father. Food was a big way of showing love and affection for my father and my paternal grandparents. Last time I visited my father's parents at their house, I remember my grandma had literally baked two cakes, three types of brownies, and five different types of cookies, and had made a couple of different puddings. I was old enough to know that that much sugary food was not good for me, but I felt guilty not eating some of the sweets, because grandma had put so much effort into making all these different confections for my sister and me. Another time when I was eight, my father took us up to Virginia to visit the grandparents for a whole week. I don't know why I was so anxious about that trip, but the whole time I was there I didn't eat. I just couldn't – every time I tried to eat, I couldn't swallow. My throat felt as though it was closing up. I didn't have an upset stomach or anything, I was just too anxious to stomach anything. My grandparents and dad thought I was sick and took me to the doctor while I was up there, but they didn't find anything wrong. In actuality, it was all in my head.

Another incident of "food paralysis" also happened with dad. It was one of his weekends with me, and he had made Sloppy Joes for dinner. Though I was still a kid in elementary school, those sandwiches just didn't look appetizing. I told him I didn't like them while dad protested that we had

had them before. I was overcome by anxiety at the idea I might be forced to eat this. My stomach churned and I went numb and tingly in my chest. I refused to eat; the very thought repulsed me. My dad was livid, and his anger frightened me. Despite a few uncomfortable hours after dinner, one of my fondest memories came later that night. I felt I was at fault for making him angry and wanted to say I was sorry. When I went out to apologize, he was reclining on the lounge chair on the porch. I sat with him and we looked at the stars in the night sky. That was the night I picked out "my star." To this day, I always reflect upon that star when I need to get lost in my thoughts.

The reason I tell these stories is because I used to look to food for comfort and as a way to fill a void in my life. Despite many very uncomfortable times dealing with food, I sought it out for comfort when I was alone. It never lasted long and turned into feelings of guilt and self-loathing. It is very easy to allow food to consume and control how we live life. I still have moments when I look to food for comfort, but I now mainly look at it as a way to fuel my body properly. Today, when I am with friends and family, food no longer controls my emotions. I use the gathering, not the food itself, to nourish my soul with memories, laughter, and meaning.

I used to think happiness would come from excelling in school, but I ended up missing out on fun group events. I used to think happiness would come from chasing a career I was passionate about, but I ended up putting other important things on the backburner. I used to think happiness would come from being skinny. What my fitness journey has taught me is that happiness does not come from WHAT I look like, but in discovering WHO I am. My journey has allowed me to define the "what" while exploring the "who." The self-discovery I have found in creating who I was meant to be all along has been the most exhilarating part of this experience. The physical transformation would not be the same without the experience of getting to know my truest self and no longer being bound by the bodily restrictions I placed on myself.

I am not sure exactly when I started to feel an overall satisfaction in the changes I was making. The sense of happiness in who I am becoming sort of snuck up on me. I see self-discovery as an ever- evolving state of being. I am far happier today than I have ever previously been. I am happier with my body. I am happier with who I am. My happiness ebbs and flows; of course, I want to find that balance where it remains constant. I didn't think falling in love with fitness and a healthy lifestyle would help me discover my authentic self, my deepest heart, and my true passions.

This self-discovery allowed me to fall in love with myself, because I realized I am not defined by my body. I have learned to value my worth in who I am becoming more than what I look like. I am not becoming skinny. I am not becoming abs. I am not becoming muscle lines. I am becoming a strong mind. I am becoming a happier heart. I am becoming a more confident soul. It truly is about synchronizing with your mind, body, heart, and spirit. I work on my body because exercise and feeling good helps my mind. Because my mind is becoming stronger and clearer, my heart is becoming softer, gentler, more open, and kinder.

The things my mind used to control are now in the domain of my heart. By relinquishing this head-centered control, my soul is gradually becoming more confident and comfortable in all that I am. I used to think a flat stomach or thin thighs would make me happier or prettier. I thought losing weight was the answer to feeling beautiful and the ultimate sign of worthiness of all the things I desired. I believed the life I wanted was only attainable by being attractive and thin. Thank goodness, I learned life is too freaking short to be caught up in my appearance. Nowadays, my happiness comes from focusing less on my appearances and more on cultivating a mind and heart that is beautiful beyond doubt.

I am still on my quest for happiness. I want to know what it will mean for me, what it will feel like, how I will define it. Will I ever truly know pure happiness? Or will it remain a figment of my imagination? Maybe happiness is not meant for me. Maybe my brain is wired to never know genuine joy because of my anxious tendencies. How do you prioritize happiness? I have learned happiness is not defined by my body or losing weight. I have weighed less than I do currently and I was still very unhappy. The problem is that happiness is not some sort of destination at which you just "arrive". But it can be found through the journey itself. I have the choice to be happy right now, in this moment, today. But that is far easier said than done most days. The practice requires thought and mindfulness in every present moment for me.

CH:9

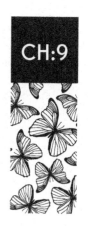

Like a Butterfly, Constantly Changing

The day after my 26th birthday I walked into my therapist's office for the first time in roughly five years and exclaimed, "I am so excited to be here!" For the next hour, I proceeded to pour out my life story to a stranger, sharing intimate details that I rarely share with anyone except those I trust implicitly. I was seven months into my new healthy lifestyle and was feeling great about myself for the first time ever. Nonetheless, pain and embarrassment from the past continued to haunt me with the fear of being emotionally vulnerable and seen for who I am and not what I look like. My mind, body, heart, and soul were coming together, yet I remained in need of meaning, connection, balance, and real harmony.

At age 16, I was very sure of everything about my future. I was not that much of a gamer, but I loved playing Zoo Tycoon for hours on the weekends. One day it hit me that there are people that actually design zoos for a living. In a flash, I realized my calling. I immediately logged out of the game I was playing and started researching a career as a zoo designer. Along the way, I also encountered the profession of landscape architecture. My mind was made up and I was determined to make this dream come true.

From a young age, I was always doing something artistic or crafty. I imagined I would end up in a creative industry. My high school art teachers constantly encouraged me to pursue a job in illustration; somehow illustration seemed to be more of a hobby to me. I was also very passionate about animal conservation. Landscape architecture was the perfect blend of art and science, and I could easily picture my future as a zoo designer. For the next seven years, I fervently pursued a degree in landscape architecture. In college, I understood I would not be a zoo designer right out of school, but I enjoyed it enough to continue to pursue my degree. As you can imagine, zoo design is a very specialized pursuit within this larger profession, but I was doggedly determined to get there. I had a few opportunities to explore the conceptual ideas of conservation intertwined with design at college, which I found very appealing. My parents weren't as convinced. My dad would ask, "Are you sure you like this profession enough to pursue it even if you are not designing zoos?" I believed it was the perfect fit for me. I knew it would take time to grow into the zoo design industry, and I had my blinders on and vision set on this achievement. This was going to happen one day. My first interview out of college was with one of the best firms in the industry. I was stoked because I knew my career would be set if I landed a job there. When I didn't get the job, I was crushed. It took five months to land a job; during the job search, I began questioning if I belonged in the industry.

At first, everything was terrific. I loved my job and my new home in Florida. But a little over a year into my career adventure, something shifted, and not for the better. I had been working on a few team projects in the production stage leading up to the Christmas season. Once we got back from our holiday break, my projects had moved out of production and my workload lightened. At this company we ran on billable hours with time assigned to specific projects. As the weeks went by, my billable hours filled less of my week. This was a pretty big issue. We conducted staff meetings every Monday, and every week I struggled to land enough work for the week. At times, I would only get about eight to sixteen hours for the forty-hour work week. It not only was a problem for my efficiency and productivity as an employee, it was a problem for my self-esteem.

I became embarrassed and felt like no one wanted to work with me. I would volunteer my time and the project would be given to someone else or my boss would say, "Are you sure you can take that on?" I would think, "Um, yes I am sure! I only have six hours scheduled for this week." Occasionally, I would land enough work but with project schedules always shifting, I would suddenly find myself without hours for the week. At one point, I was asked to do a quick sketch, exciting yet a bit of a challenge for me. I had not had an opportunity to draw in quite some time but gave it my best effort. After producing the sketch, I ended up overhearing my managers' reaction to it. Unbeknownst to the manager and the project manager, I was just at the right distance and angle to see them reviewing it. Their reaction was devastating to witness. It took a full week before the project manager who assigned the task reviewed it with me to explain what was wrong, how it could have been corrected, and how I should have approached the task differently.

I started feeling uncomfortable at work; I had to constantly send out emails or ask project managers if they needed help with anything. I would go to my main project manager seeking assignments, she was supposed to be my mentor, but she was cold, distant, and unapproachable. I shied away from approaching her with questions on how I could become a better team member. The message was that I did not belong.

I began to question if I was somehow being set up for failure. I knew I needed a change. Out of the blue I received an email from another local landscape architect asking if I was looking for a change. It could not have come at a better time. In spite of this, I was terrified to explore the opportunity and ignored it for about a month until I had no choice but to make a change. I was worried the opportunity might be been long gone, but I still gave it a try. I needed to for my sanity.

Sure enough, there was still an opening, but it came with a lot of risk. I would be going to a smaller firm, something I had never thought I wanted. I would be working with a newer, less established company and would have to take a pay cut. Despite having just bought a house a few months earlier with a mortgage to cover, I ultimately decided my happiness and mental health was far more important than anything else. I knew I needed to make the change to avoid total self-destruction.

Saying goodbye to my first job after college was a lot harder than I anticipated. Despite how miserable it made me, I still had an attachment to the place and the people. But for a long time, I blamed the people at my old job for how I felt about myself. It took many months, almost a year in fact, for me to learn to forgive. The forgiveness was not about how I felt others had treated me, the forgiveness was for myself. I constantly berated myself with messages like, "You are not good enough. You are not worthy. You are talentless and never were truly creative." I learned that sometimes the negativity we feel others place upon us is really coming from within. Yes, there were external forces driving these feelings. But I had a choice. I could have chosen to be better for myself and stood up for myself across the board. Or I could choose to run away from those feelings and not face those emotional challenges. I chose to run away. I knew the change was the right move for me and my sense of self. Every day we are faced with hundreds of choices that can alter our future, but with those decisions come both the choice and power to change.

The job change was an interesting transition, to say the least. I went from working with 20 plus people, many of whom were young, to working with three middle-aged men. Very quickly though I realized that the change was worth the risk. Within just a few weeks, I felt happier and more worthy. I was working on cool, fun, and exciting projects. I was doing more design and less construction documentation. I felt a creative spark and realized I had not lost all my artistic abilities. I felt more energized and excited and passionate about life again. I got to go to the Bahamas on a site visit just a few weeks in. I got to be a lead designer on a new project being built. I was feeling so much better, but something was still absent. There is always a missing puzzle piece or two, and those pieces were happiness, connection, and meaning.

For so long, I let the fear of change and the fear of the unknown dictate my life. I took a psychology class in college; without a doubt, it was my favorite class. I used to say if landscape architecture didn't work out, I would have been a therapist. That should have been my sign, but I felt utterly committed to the idea of designing zoos and the degree I had worked so hard to get.

About a month after starting my new job, I began my fitness journey and my Instagram account @plankingforpizza. I had no idea whatsoever how meaningful and impactful this decision would be. About seven or eight months into my new job, the "honeymoon phase" of happiness began to fade. Stress and anxiety began to pick up. My fitness journey took on more importance and become more meaningful and passionate. I noticed my happiness level was changing, not because of my job and not because of my changing body. It was simply because my idea of myself was changing. Every part of my being as I knew it was completely changing. My body was undergoing physical changes, which helped in contributing to growing happiness and confidence, but my mindset and my heart were also developing significantly. My job began to seem less important; there was no connection I yearned for. My meaning and connection was definitely elsewhere.

That trip to the therapist's office was a turning point. I was changing, but I was not sure what was happening. After a month or so of therapy, I began to understand what was going on. I had placed so much of the basis of my happiness in what I was doing with my life and the idealized career I was chasing. I had been raised to be very independent, goal-oriented, and career driven. Now, this career path did not feel right for me. For so long, I felt that I was defined by my career. So much so that in a way, I lost touch with my own identity. I was no longer "Jess, the girl with the weird obsessions with designing zoos." I had been that girl for almost 10 years. It was scary giving that girl up.

A lot of my anxiety stems from simply being overwhelmed with life and what goals to tackle first, and how to deal with everyday stresses and pressures, both those placed on me by others and those I place on myself. My therapist often reminds me, "You are *so* hard on yourself." And I know she is right. I am very hard on myself as a result of the sense of unworthiness and inadequacy I picked up as a child. That is the little girl within me coming to the surface. The past is something we can never change, yet all along I have been trying to change my past, while also trying to understand it and searching for answers for why things happened the way they did. I have allowed myself to settle into the comfort of the discomfort of my current situation.

Our everyday choices lead to change. We have the choice to work out or not. We have the choice to eat healthy or eat a whole pizza. We have a choice, to settle for our circumstances or to free ourselves from self-imprisonment. I have several big choices in my future, and many of them involve big changes. It is scary, but I know it will be worth it. Without doubt, the happiness I have been searching for is on the other side of change. Recently I have found that I must allow myself to keep changing and becoming more comfortable with the unknown. But it can be terrifying, it can make me want to crawl into a hole. But that is the old me talking. The new me knows better. The new me understands that self-improvement and betterment are a continuum. Every day that we wake up, we are provided with an abundance of gifts, and one of our greatest gifts is the ability to choose. We can choose to settle for misery or we can choose self-improvement.

Self-improvement is not just physical, it is also mental and emotional. You can be content with your body, but you may still not be happy. I have discovered my happiness has nothing to do with my body. I have learned any happiness I will ever have lies in what I do and who I become. I have learned I do not want my success in life to be mine alone; my best successes in life are through the successes of others. Once again, change is on the horizon. How this change is going to happen? I am still figuring that out as I write this book.

I allowed fear of change to keep me from evolving into a better me. I was afraid to work out and eat right because I thought my results and efforts would never be good enough. I was afraid I still would not be happy with myself, or that I would not be any more attractive or worthy of the things I desired. I was afraid to change jobs because I thought I would end up in a place that might even be worse. Nevertheless, I made a decision for change. Not all of the changes have been positive, but that is how we learn, that is how we grow. Change, whether good or bad, always leads to some personal development, because we learn from both the negative and positive. Change might be intimidating when it presents itself, but if it feels right, DO IT! Even if it feels wrong, maybe there is an unforeseen reason why a possibility has presented itself. You don't have to jump in feet first, but you owe it to yourself to explore the opportunity. Don't wait until you need to; do it because you want to.

For so long, I felt as though I was a caterpillar, so unsure of the future or what my evolution would look like. I still feel that way sometimes. The beautiful thing about the caterpillar is that it does not question the transformation itself, it just goes through metamorphosis. Beauty is not about appearances, it is about the journey and the changes that make us evolve into the fullness of ourselves. I am still learning to trust the change with confidence and commitment. Sometimes we progress forwards and other times we go backwards. It is okay to question as you go. Questioning ourselves, our potential, and our happiness is what helps us grow and develop into who we are meant to become. There is nothing worse than remaining the same and not seeking your fullest potential simply because of fear of failure and self-doubt through the process of change. I have changed for the worse and I have changed for the better. What I know for sure is that taking a chance on change, even in the darkest of times, allows our butterfly to emerge.

Change Challenge

It is always important to conduct self inquiry. Ask yourself: how can I improve as an individual? This challenge is simple. It is about setting goals, both large and small, for changes you want in your life. Maybe you want to lose 10 pounds or maybe you want to do something big like learn to love yourself or chase a new dream. Whatever your goal may be, it is a great idea to diagram and visualize the change(s) you would like. Try this art challenge: draw out a butterfly. Remember, this is not about being the most artistic person and drawing the perfect butterfly. It is ok if it looks like a two-year old drew it, because it is the message it will carry on its wings that is most important and beautiful of all. This is not about appearance, but about meaning. On the body of the butterfly, write out the change you wish to make. If you have a few changes you wish to make, draw one butterfly per change. Take care to not overwhelm the one butterfly with many changes. This butterfly, or series of butterflies if you have a few changes you wish to make, will represent endurance, hope, and revitalization of your soul by representing the changes you wish to see. Change can be burdensome and weigh us down mentally and emotionally. I hope by writing out a plan and visually seeing the effective changes you wish to make these little drawings can literally and figuratively "carry the weight" for you. Next, on the wings of the butterfly, list out two to three action plans or goals you can set that will help you achieve that big picture change. Simply writing these things out will not create this change. Taking action will bring about. These butterflies symbolize your acceptance of transformation. Embrace the changes you wish to make and chase those dreams with elegance, grace, and faith as you undergo this metamorphosis.

If you wish to share your drawings on Instagram or Twitter, use hash tag #butterflychangechallenge and tag me in your picture so I can see!

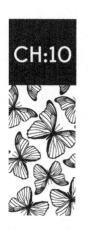

Compassion over Comparison

CH:10

I often wonder how different I may be today had social media been as big of an influence as it is today when I was younger. During those vulnerable middle school years, the internet as we use it today was not in such common use. Facebook had only just begun but I did not know about it until many years later. Instagram was far in the future. I was on MySpace but I did not use it often. Even though I did not have many online influences, magazines were everywhere with headlines like: "Real women are curvy: how to enhance those curves," "How to lose 10 pounds in one month," "Get flat abs fast," "Tips to make you look beautiful," or "How to get a bangin' body." Image after image, all pictures of "that perfect body" I felt I could never achieve.

It was hard to know what was acceptable in terms of appearances. At the time I probably was mostly concerned with that article on "How to get that perfectly crimped hair", yet browsing those magazines still left me feeling inadequate because of all the articles about having a "perfect body." I constantly compared myself to the girls around me and often thought I was not enough because I was not skinny or pretty like the girls in magazines or even in my school. I think I spent most of my youth and young adult years comparing myself to others. I always wanted to be skinny, or popular, or pretty, or have their clear skin, or their expensive designer clothes. I wanted to be just like them. I wanted to be someone other than me.

My worst years were those spent in high school. I don't remember comparing myself to others before middle school; I had not yet been socialized about what was deemed beautiful or what was considered average or inadequate in terms of appearance. After I quit gymnastics, I still wanted to do something active that would help me maintain my flexibility and tumbling skills. The only other activity I could think of that would accomplish this was cheerleading. From eighth grade through my senior year of high school I was a cheerleader. I was not a competitive sport cheerleader, because the stunt aspect terrified me. I was a sideline cheerleader for the basketball and football teams at school.

I had some great times as a cheerleader, but I also had some really unhappy times as well. I was rarely a favorite because I was uncomfortably shy. I failed to stand out. Yet I had tumbling and coordination skills that seemed to be on my side during tryouts. I had always hoped cheerleading would help me break out of my shell. Unfortunately, the opposite happened. In tenth grade, I had made the JV football and Varsity basketball cheer squads. Many girls from my freshman year had made the Varsity football squad, so I felt left out that I did not also make that Varsity football team as well. I was one of two sophomores on the JV squad, everyone else was a freshman. It was a great learning opportunity and could have been an even better leadership experience. I was confident I was going to become a co-captain with the other sophomore girl because it made sense for the two sophomores to be the captains. When this didn't happen, I was devastated. I was the odd one out; all the freshman and sophomore girls all knew each other from attending the same middle school. I believe our coach should have stepped in and changed that outcome, but I was not assertive enough. I could have been a better role model for some of the freshman girls, but instead I resented trying out for the football squad. I wanted nothing more than to quit. Forfeiting my position on the JV football squad would have meant sacrificing my position on the Varsity basketball squad. I stuck with it as best as I could. Nothing made me feel more inadequate than not being a squad captain that season.

That season I started being more sensitive about my body. I had terrible *bacne* during middle and high school. The tank tops we often had to wear would always show acne outbreaks, which me feel really insecure. No one else on the team seemed to suffer with *bacne* like I had. I was not the smallest girl on the squad, but just like in gymnastics, I was built different. Looking through old photos, I was by no means overweight or fat, but I still could not help but feel as though I was too big to be on the team. I remember one distinct conversation at practice. One of the girls, as it happened the other sophomore on my squad, kept remarking on my behind: "Your butt is so big," she would say and other girls would chime in. I felt targeted and I equated "big" with "fat." I responded in such an embarrassing way. I got defensive and said something along the lines of, "Quit saying my butt is big, or you are going to make me do bad things," meaning that I was going to not eat and try to starve myself so that I would lose my big butt. That was a bit dramatic in the way of a response, but in that moment, I felt desperate. The conversation ended, but I was left feeling even more insecure.

After my sophomore year, I only tried out for the basketball team. The girls on the football squad were different than the girls on the basketball squad. I felt more welcomed that year on the basketball squad than I did with the football girls. I looked up to some of the older girls,and since I was the youngest, many of them began to look out for me. That probably was the best cheerleading squad and season I experienced! Sophomore cheerleading season started poorly but ended on a great note. Things started to decline again once I was a junior and senior, because most of the older friends I admired had graduated.

Girls at this age can be all drama and cattiness; cheerleading was no exception. Even the cheer moms could start things. Looking back, I can see it was ridiculous. I remember a total Mean Girl moment that happened when I had a sleepover at my house with the squad. I spent all day baking and making truffles for the girls, something I loved to do. One of the girls said, "Next time we need to do this at a house that is bigger and more comfortable." It was so hurtful to be defined by what I did or didn't have. Maybe I didn't grow up in the biggest house, but I am thankful for that, because my parents were able to afford fun trips that made for wonderful memories. I considered the concept of popularity based on living in a better neighborhood with bigger houses. I had no say in what house I grew up in or where. This comment was more than just a stab at me, it was a slam aimed at my family.

High school was a bit of a rough time for me, as it was for many people. Problems at home caused me to act out. I was never the rebellious type. I did well in school, avoided parties, and rarely got in trouble, but I would allow my emotions to get in the way of my interactions with others. I tried not to involve myself in any drama, but sometimes it was inevitable. At the time, I had a problematic relationship with my biological father. I would go months without talking with him; I asked him not to come to the games where I was cheering. He would show up unexpectedly and I would remove myself to the sidelines to calm my nerves and anxiety. Without going into all the details, (my family history could be a whole another book on its own, but for now, I won't go there,) I was afraid of my dad. I can't really explain why because I honestly don't know. There may be suppression I hold on to that keeps me from remembering. Part of me wants to understand my past better, but another part wants to keep moving forward. My relationship with him has been on the mend for a few years now.

My most destructive thoughts would surface when my dad showed up unannounced. I took my stress out on the other girls because I did not know how to handle my feelings. As result, many of the girls seemed a little disconnected from me. For away games, I would be sitting alone on the bus or with the food for the game. I would try to join in with conversations happening around me, but it was not always easy. I would sit low in my seat with my music, me alone with my thoughts. It is weird feeling so alone while being surrounded by so many people.

139

It was disheartening to not have anyone want to sit with me most of the time. I always felt like there was something wrong with me or that I was unlikeable. I am only just now starting to connect all these dots. I could have been more liked. I could have been more outgoing. I could have been less sensitive. I could have been friendlier. But I wasn't, because I didn't know how to separate home from school. Instead I broke down and drowned in the shallow pit of comparison. I allowed myself to be defined by how others treated me. In reality, I needed to learn how to treat myself better.

In college, I would get jealous of other girls I thought were prettier than me. College was a rough time for me; the family issues didn't go away. I figured the only way I could help out my family was to excel in school. That's exactly what I did, and I did so with comparison. My art classes and art teacher were my safe haven in high school. I went to college well prepared with a strong design sense and creative background. I pursued a degree in landscape architecture, which is a creative/design field. Many of my peers did not have the artistic background I had, so I began to compare myself in that way. Grades were subjective because art is subjective. I always wanted to have the best design and best illustrative graphics (though I was not the best), so when other students would get better grades or have better designs than I did, I yet again often deemed myself to be lacking. Art was my talent. It was how I excelled in high school. It was my way of expressing myself emotionally without actually using words. Art was my freedom.

Landscape architecture is a creative industry, but it can be artistically limiting. There are budgets, client preferences, and location constraints that must be kept in mind, so I don't feel the same sense of originality working in this profession as when I am painting. In school, we frequently had the same site design, and there was always a critique comparing your work with other students' work. I get that constructive criticism is important for growth, but I also critiqued my work internally and compared myself with my peers. If one of my designs failed, and anything less than an A was a failure to me, I was distraught.

These are just some of the ways I have been caught up in comparison. Prior to starting my fitness journey, I would send "fitspo" images to my roommate: "This body is my goal" or "I want to look like her." I still have a tendency to compare, but now it is my lifestyle that I compare with what I see online. I want what "they" have. The truth is, I can't have what they have, because their dreams and goals are not my own. The best I have learned to do is stop comparing what I want with what others have. This set me back in the past because I lost motivation to move forward. It is hard to know what others are going through. What people post online tends to be a "highlight reel" of life. That is exactly why I show my good and bad sides. I have found that cheering others on in their successes and compassion for their failures has significantly helped me along the way.

It took about eight ***** into my own journey for me to discover this point of view. Now I rarely look at others girls and say, "I want what she has." There is no way to sugar coat this – SHE is not ME, and it is as simple as that. Compassion is about giving, it is not about getting. Sometimes it is hard to be happy for other's successes when they are not reciprocating that happiness for your successes. When staying true to myself, my heart, and my mind, it doesn't affect me as much. I feel better if I feel happy for other's successes instead of letting jealousy, envy, or insecurity get the best of me.

Somewhere in the mess of it all, this just clicked. I needed to just own my own life and my own sense of beauty. I began to really take note of the influence I had on others through my pictures and messages. People picked up on this change as well. Some shied away because I seemed a little different, but many more began to take note of how I began to show up in a truer light. I stopped comparing myself to an external ideal by trying to post only the best pictures of my body. I stopped comparing myself by being open about my struggles with anxiety and seeing a therapist. I was open, raw, and vulnerable about my mental health struggles and how that impacted my poor body image. To me, mental health is not talked about enough in our society. I believe it is important to start being more honest about it since so many people struggle silently, thinking they are alone with their negative and self-loathing thoughts. The more I open up and share, the more girls open up to me and say they feel the same. So many women deal with body insecurity and poor self-image. I am sure it has to do with the influence of society and impact of media. Many are afraid to open up and talk about their internal struggles because of the stigma associated with depression. There is nothing wrong with needing help or admitting your struggle. Often people are afraid to admit anything because they risk being judged as "crazy" when this is rarely the case. Just know that you are not your mental illness, just as you are not body fat, you are not cellulite, you are not acne, and mostly importantly: you are not alone. I stopped making negative comparisons of myself, my body, and my life by giving myself permission to be me.

There have been moments where I have thought, "This is too embarrassing. Why would I share this?" or "Do people like the real me?"   I remind myself how important it is to stay true to myself, because I know my authenticity is what's most important to share and that this connects me more deeply with others. There are so many expectations about and standards of body image in today's world; and I find by showing my body in more natural states, it is more liberating than showing myself at my best. I feel less pressure to be some "perfect" expression that I showcase online. The most rewarding and reassuring moments are when younger girls reach out to me and tell me they feel better or more confident about themselves because I often show what they call the "less than the societal ideal" aspects of my body. I no longer feel caught up in comparison when these moments happen, because I know I am owning my truest self. Nothing has been more liberating!

As I have grown mentally on my journey, I have come to realize that comparison is simply a mask. I used to never allow my truest self to shine through. Comparison always fails to make me feel any better about myself. I began to really embrace my individuality right around my year mark, because I was no longer striving to be someone I never could be. All my life I have been living by other's standards and trying to please those around me or be who others wanted me to be. When I stopped chasing a life that was not my own, I began to live my life as it was designed by me. It is so very easy to get caught up in a web of comparison and self-doubt, especially with how prevalent social media is today in our lives. I have frequently made comparisons of both my body and my life. I still catch myself doing so when I'm down. It has made me wonder why I am not cool enough to do amazing things, or why I am not courageous enough to step outside my comfort zone. I learned though that by comparing not just my body, but my life, to those of others, I lose my individuality in the process.

I have learned that by surrendering comparison and embracing compassion, I am now able to allow my truth to fully emerge. This in turn allows my mind to be more honest, my heart to be more vulnerable, and my soul to feel less restricted. My authentic self has emerged from learning more about who I am and not allowing myself to compare my worth to that of others. One of my favorite analogies is what they say about snowflakes: no two are exactly alike. And that is just how bodies, personalities, individuals, and lives are. No two are exactly the same, nor should they be. The girls I used to look at in envy because they had "perfect" bodies or lives, I now look at in compassion and admiration, because I can only imagine what has gone into crafting this life they live. Mostly, I now recognize that there is so much power in being able to own who YOU are. My greatest gift in self-love was to stop wanting to be someone I am not and can never be. I learned that I had to own who I am, what I look like, and what my life is like. If I do not like something, I have the power to change, BUT ONLY IF it fits into chasing the dreams, life, and body that I desire and know are right for me and only me. There is not a "one size fits all" to looks or to life. It truly looks different on everyone!

Create a Compassion Compass

I will admit it can be difficult being happy for other's successes. Jealousy and envy can control not just how we treat others, but ourselves as well. It is easy to be envious of someone who lost 50 pounds and has sky-high self-esteem as a result, or of someone who may have just landed their ultimate dream job.In the past it has been so very easy for me to belittle others and say, "They did not deserve that success," when I was really wondering, "Why have I not found that same success? I must be inadequate and unworthy of such achievement." I have found that by genuinely being happy for or praising the unique qualities of others, even though it can be difficult to do, I end up feeling better about myself because I am not lost in the comparison trap.

For this exercise, I want you to envision what compassion looks like for yourself and others. I think it would be great if you can create a **"compassion compass"** that expresses empathy and maps out how you can more easily be compassionate.

Creativity should not be limited; this can look however you envision it. I love the symbolism behind a compass. To me, the image of the compass represents unity, direction, discovery, and guidance. Your directional forces do not have to be North, South, East or West. They could be Positivity, Grace, Acceptance, Kindness, etc. You don't have to be limited to four compass points; this is an exercise for you and what you want to work on. Whatever you need to discover, I want you to craft a representation that will best guide you toward more compassion for yourself and others. This will enable you to stop comparing yourself to others so you can live your purpose in a compassionate manner.

I would love to see your compassion compass and how you chose to express yourself through this exercise. If you feel inclined to share on Instagram or Twitter, please use hashtag #compassioncompass and tag me in the photo so I can see what you create.

Perfectionism

When I moved to Florida some years ago, I saw this as an opportune time to reinvent myself. I didn't have a traditional college experience because of the "good girl mentality" I carried with me from childhood. I look back now and see that frame of mind prevented a lot of self-discovery. I did not go out much, nor did I party. My first taste of alcohol only occurred after my 21st birthday. I always stayed up late working on projects and studying. Before relocating to Florida, I told myself, "Now is my time to shine! To truly allow myself to be the outgoing, fun-loving, loud, me!" What I failed to realize was how difficult and uncomfortable that could be. My shyness constrained my ability to fully be me. I did not have anyone to shine for or to shine with. I simply had my dog, my cat, and myself.

The day after college graduation, I headed down to South Florida for my first interview with my only job prospect; it was with a prestigious firm for my profession. I was honored to be selected for this interview. I was incredibly excited;

my career could be set. After two telephone interviews and two days of in-person interviews followed by a three week wait, everything came crashing to a halt. I didn't get the job. I was crushed. For a few days, I was in a state of complete panic, since this was my only potential job offer. I had been confident that I would get it. When I didn't get hired, I felt utterly unworthy for a job in my chosen profession. What could I do? Were there any other jobs available? There were so many unknowns and so much trepidation. I took everything personally.

Finances dictated that I had to leave the college town I had grown to love and move back home to my parents'. Five years gone in the blink of an eye. What did I truly know? Who had I actually become? I had put so much time and effort into my studies that I had not allowed myself to live the typical college life. Here I was a college graduate with an accredited five-year degree, no job prospects, and no plans for the future. The future I had envisioned for myself at age 16 was now lost. It seemed that I had been on track to a goal that would never be realized. Even worse, while chasing that dream, I had forgotten to truly live.

The months after graduation were a tough transition for me. I bounced back and forth between my mom's house and my dad's house, searching for what to do with myself. In college, I found myself a cat, but there were already two cats at mom's house. I spent my days at my dad's house visiting with my cat and searching for a job. I spent countless hours sending out emails and resumes, hoping someone, somewhere, anywhere, would have an entry-level job opening. Rejection after rejection poured in and this started to bring me down. I began to think there was no hope for a future in my chosen profession; I questioned whether I should start looking elsewhere. My inner 16-year old was determined to not give up on this dream.

Three months after graduation, I was still stuck with no job prospects. Not the best time for my life to get a little more complicated. On the way home from a long family visit in Tennessee, we were taking back roads in the north Georgia Mountains when I witnessed something a little heartbreaking. We crossed an intersection and passed a car parked on the side of the road there. As we drove by, I noticed a little pup in the tall grasses beside the car. Once we cleared the intersection, the parked car sped through the intersection as this tiny pup chased after the car. It was one of the saddest things I ever witnessed. We figured the puppy had just been abandoned; I didn't have it in my heart to leave him behind. Dad was driving and maybe made it a quarter mile before my pleas and cries convinced him to turn around. When we got back, the puppy was nowhere to be seen. When we stopped, my dad's girlfriend gets out and starts calling, "Puppy, puppy, puppy!" After a couple of minutes, the floppy-eared little fellow comes bounding out of the tall grass. He was so precious. Upon first inspection, he showed signs of neglect; he was covered in fleas and ticks with reddened eyes. He was such a sweetie; we simply could not leave him behind.

As we pull away, dad asks, "Ok, so now what?"

His girlfriend replies, "We need to name him!"

Startled, I responded with, "We cannot name him. If we do, that means we are keeping him and he is mine. I cannot have a dog right now."

149 🐾

Long story short, we named him Coosa after the river where we found him. He has turned out to be the biggest blessing and the biggest pain in my ass ever since that moment. I am tearing up as I recount this story;   I cannot fathom not having this dog in my life. I do believe everything happens for a reason. There's a reason I didn't get that first job. There's a reason I didn't find a job for months. There's a reason I took time to visit family that weekend. And there is definitely a reason I was there in that moment to witness my future dog being abandoned. I didn't rescue my dog; Coosa rescued me. Another man's trash certainly became my biggest treasure.

A few weeks after finding Coosa, I ended up landing a job with a great firm in Central Florida. I had always pictured myself moving out west. Florida wasn't in my plans. Yet again, everything happens for a reason. I was ready to begin my new life, so I went for it! It was intimidating moving to a new state where I didn't know a soul. Still, it was an exciting adventure and I was ready to reinvent myself. I never imagined that with reinvention would also come total self-destruction.

In the beginning, I was doing great. I was feeling good about my job and myself. I walked my very energetic pup three miles every day. I was fortunate to have Coosa as protection and as a valued companion. I immensely enjoyed spending time with him outside. I loved the weather and new scenery, and everything seemed a good fit. And it was all pretty perfect until it wasn't. It took a long, long time for Florida to feel like home. I didn't make new friends immediately, so it became a little lonely. As winter in Florida approached, I walked Coosa less often and would end up "eating my feelings" on nights and weekends. The terrible eating habits I picked up in college escalated. Pretty much every weekend was filled with devouring entire pizzas, whole boxes of cereal, or family-sized bags of chips in one sitting in front of the TV. You know the saying, "What you eat in private, you wear in public"? That quickly became my reality. I had no idea what real loneliness could be.

It took about eight months before I met my roommate, who is now my best friend. I believe certain people come into our lives when we least expect it, and my roommate happened to be one of those people. It was eerie how similar we were; we had more similarities in values, morals, and upbringing than differences. I swore she could have been a sister from a past life. She was unlike any of my other friends and began to challenge me in a good way.

There was something so appealing about her. She reminded me somewhat of a dear friend from college who had been a great comfort. I admired the way she could captivate a crowd. I longed for her outgoing, friendly spirit and lived vicariously through her. I wanted to be like her – pretty, fit, and with an infectious personality. I observed from the sidelines in order to "learn her ways." Watching her failed to yield the confidence I craved, leaving me with the sense that I was destined to be on the sidelines. She sparkled with a commanding attitude and witty brilliance. Above all, she came off as comfortable, content, and self-assured. Of course, she isn't without insecurities; she simply does not allow them to rule her life in the same way that I had. Through her friendship, I concluded I needed to get comfortable in my own skin, which was easier said than done.

After a few months, we decided to become roommates. I intended to not live with anyone else until I got married, but the positives outweighed the negatives. This was far and away the best decision I had made since moving to Florida. My roommate was into fitness and helped me start to clean up my eating habits by teaching me a thing or two about nutrition. We started going to the gym together and established a pretty good routine. Before moving in together, I had begun to consider becoming a first-time home buyer. I had put in an offer the day before she asked to be roommates. I wanted to make many improvements on the home first before moving in, so for several months I shuttled between apartment and house. It didn't take long before I fell out of my good routine and back into old habits. Things were changing, and not for the better.

My "quarter life crisis" was just beginning. Soon, it was going full force – I questioned my talents, , my work ethic, and my motivation. Every notion of my being was in question. I had always had a good work ethic and level of motivation. I knew I was talented and creative, yet I was falling apart. I began to feel unworthy. I cast about in despair, trying to find myself again. This is when I started drinking, heavily, desperate for answers. Alcohol had never been a part of my life until now. I had sworn it off and was proud that it wasn't a part of my life. In college, not drinking gave me my own kind of independence from the social norm. But strangely, in this dark time I yearned for it. Not alcohol itself, but how I felt while consuming it, free and uninhibited, reckless and uncontrollable. Here was that outgoing, life-of-the-party girl I knew that I was deep down. "Rebelling" against my morals created an uncomfortable chasm between my heart and mind, a dark secret I kept in order to protect my family. I thought drinking would help me feel again, and to an extent, it did. Just not in a healthy way. The "let loose" feeling was something I didn't want to let go of. I liked not caring what others thought; releasing all my insecurities and shyness was liberating. Despite the destruction, I finally allowed myself to be imperfect. Somehow, in this damaged time, I finally allowed myself to see my true self.

Honestly, imperfection is a wonderful revelation. A part of me was reluctant to give up the confidence I felt while drinking. But I knew it was not a habit to keep. The shift from perfectionist to realist came at exactly the right time. I released the feelings of inadequacy and realized that I deserved better; I chose to rise above the despair and self-destruction.

My perfectionism might have stemmed from being the oldest child with a need to please. Ever since I can remember, I always had to be "perfect." I placed pressure on myself to be the best I could be in everything I did: school, sports, extracurricular activities, artistic endeavors, everything. I placed a lot of emphasis on my appearance. I was not the prettiest, the skinniest, or the most popular girl growing up. But I never gave credit to the worth of my mind and heart; as an awkward teenager, I placed all my value in my looks.

While rarely a "perfect" child, I was a pretty good kid who didn't act out, maintained good grades, gained admission into an amazing university and graduated magna cum laude, and then got an awesome first job. I did everything "by the book" for a career-oriented woman. When things started going south at the job, I crumbled under my own lack of self-worth. I lost the part of myself I had built up for so long. I no longer recognized my own reflection. In that moment, the notion of perfection no longer worked for me. I was not perfect. Life was not perfect. Life was actually really freaking hard for reasons I didn't understand. I thought it was all on me. I unraveled. I began to drown and when I lost sight of the shore, I was terrified. I had rested so much of my identity on career and profession that I didn't know who I was without that ideal. When I realized that the profession no longer fit me, I felt that I myself did not fit. I had lost the dream that had been defining me for so long. This was when I realized it is fine not to be perfect or have life completely figured out. I embraced that feeling and never looked back. I relished the new opportunity I had to learn about my real identity; finding myself in the imperfect would only lead to magnificence.

I did not change careers at this time, but ended up moving on to a new job within the same profession, hopeing to reignite the passion I had lost. But mostly I viewed this transition as the right time to work on all of me. I thought I would find happiness again by getting into shape; I was right and wrong about that, but that is another story... Ultimately I needed to find my confidence again and learn to be comfortable in my own skin. I began to view imperfection as a blessing. Being imperfect meant I could only improve, and there was a constant excitement revolving around this idea of self-improvement. I was curious how I could grow and become anew.

Experiencing everything that happened allowed me to drop the idea of perfection. This helped me go into my fitness journey with a realistic mentality. I was no longer striving to be perfect. Dropping the idea of achieving "perfection" allowed me to redirect my thoughts and goals to what I wanted and could realistically accomplish. "Why do you always feel like you need to prove you are not perfect?" a dear friend asks me sometimes, a question I still have difficulty answering. Partly it is because I have embraced imperfect as my new normal. I have grown fond of my foibles, because they led me to my strengths. In the online world that is social media, we are often plagued with images of "perfect" and highlight reels of how life and physical looks should be. I often receive comments on posts that my body or "body goals" are "perfect", and that makes me pretty uncomfortable. When I do meet people in real life, there is a preconceived notion of how I should look in person. Images online do not necessarily convey what I see in my reflection. This is why I demonstrate my flaws and imperfections to avoid any assumption I have a "perfect" body, because I don't.

I always strive to show my good, bad, and all the rest, because I don't want to create the impression or an unrealistic expectation of a "perfect" journey or transformation. I want girls to feel empowered to own their unique and beautiful body as they are today; I want them to know perfection is a body standard will never be met. You may have an idea of what your "perfect" body is, but if you always strive to match others, you'll never be satisfied because her "perfection" is NOT your "perfection." Proving I'm not perfect is a way of expressing realism. Perfectionism is not real, so why strive for something unachievable?

What have I found to be true and real? It is so very simple: LOVE! Learning to love yourself, imperfections, flaws, and all, leads to self-acceptance. This inner appreciation is what lays the foundation for change. Self-improvement is built on love, not a pursuit of false ideals. The foundation of love I have built for myself came out of darkness and uncertainty. Learning to love my perfectly imperfect self did not happen overnight. It took months. It took complete and total surrender. I unraveled to my core so that I could truly let light in to touch my soul, bringing with it warmth necessary to self-acceptance. I accepted the fact that I have fat, but I am not fat. I have made mistakes, but I am not a mistake. I have felt unworthy, but I am enough as I am. My imperfections drive me to improve, not to become perfect. I learned to accept my "societal imperfections." While loving the things I want to change is still hard, I have learned to love my heart and mind. That was easy. Are my heart and mind perfect? No. Nonetheless, they are no longer constrained or blinded by an unrealistic notion of perfection. I have never been more confident or more comfortable in my skin; this only came about when I abandoned the idea of perfection. My heart and mind are my favorite parts of me. My soul feels more complete after having been set free from the self-imprisonment that is perfectionism.

I'm Perfectly Me Project

The concept of perfectionism can be a good thing. I think there are often times and places where it is acceptable. But when it comes to a positive body image mindset, to me perfectionism has no place. It is so easy to become consumed with "fitspo" and "perfect body goals" online. I worry that it can be harmful to seek an idea of perfection by setting out to look like others who in your mind are perfect. By disconnecting from the idea of looking like someone else, I was better able to appreciate how my body began to morph towards what's appropriate for me.

I think it is detrimental to strive for perfection through the eyes of others. I hear girls saying they "won't amount to anything" because of how they are seen through the eyes of others. Family members can unintentionally place the burden of being "perfect" on us, with unmet expectations leading to a feeling of failure. All of this can be extremely harmful to self-acceptance and esteem levels. Growing up, I received insulting comments about my appearance. Either my hair was never good enough, or my clothes were too cheap. From an early age, I began to associate my worth with my appearance. When I failed to meet the expectations of others, it began to chip away at my sense of self.

To have a body-positive mindset, you must relinquish the idea of doing fitness and health perfectly. "Imperfect" CAN be successful too. It wasn't easy, but I learned to let go of that. Step by step, I developed the following concepts about expectations in my journey; this helped me to foster an environment for realistic personal goals. Contemplate and journal on the following:

Managing Expectations Journal Exercise:

○ What expectations do you feel others place on you? Do you meet them? Exceed them? Fall short? How does it impact you mentally?

○ What expectations have you placed on yourself? Are they realistic? Are they based on what others have said to you? Or are they personal?

○ Do you consider yourself a perfectionist? How so? What things could you learn to accept as imperfect? Is it about physical defects? Personality flaws? Are these things you can change?

○ If yes, why do you feel the need to change? Why do these things need to be "perfect" or even different? What establishes the criteria of "perfect" for these things?

○ If no, how have you cultivated this view of "imperfect"? And how can you embrace "imperfect" in other areas of your life?

Create An I'm Imperfectly Me Vision Board

Utilizing the prompts above, I want you to create a vision board that is based on realistic expectations on how YOU can best live a healthy, happy, body positive lifestyle. It is easy to get caught up saving images of "fitspiration," but I want you to create a vision board that is right for *you*. I want you to do some soul-searching on what is ideal yet realistic for you in terms of body image, fitness routine, and how you can comfortably accommodate a healthy eating schedule. I do not necessarily want you to find other women or girls to compare yourself to; it will be far more impactful if you can use YOURSELF as your own motivation. Take images of your favorite and least favorite qualities. Write what you love and what you can improve. Avoid using terms like "I hate this" or "I want to get rid of that" and instead try to use a language of positivity so you learn to embrace the flawlessly imperfect you. I hope this board can help you see more of who you are. I do not want you to focus on what your body is or isn't; focus on the WHO of your being and what you give to the life you are living. Try to work on building better character, not simply on improving your exterior. Once I got to know my WHO a little bit better, my thoughts and negativity about the WHAT began to dissolve. That is my hope for you in this project. Remember, you are a limited edition, own it, rock it, embrace it, and love it!

I would love to see your vision boards, so if you feel courageous enough to share, use hashtag #Imperfectlymeproject

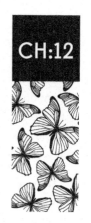

CH:12

Finding Yourself

Growing up in Georgia, I never felt a sense of belonging. I always knew Florida would not be a forever home, but of late my sense of belonging is dwindling here as well. So if not Georgia, if not Florida, where? I am wondering if maybe belonging is not a place. Maybe belonging is joining with another's heart. Or maybe belonging is with living your life as you are supposed to with passion and meaning. Or maybe it is belonging with myself. The loneliness I felt a year ago resurfaced, and I needed a break from too much solitude, from lack of belonging. Being solitary can shut me down to the point where I begin to stop receiving energy and allowing myself to be open. In these moments, alone with my thoughts, I can begin to define myself and recognize what I want out of life. I never thought my fitness journey would bring me to the greatest gift, the gift of knowing, finding, loving, and belonging to myself.

It is March 26, 2016, at 2:30 in the morning and my alarm goes off. I easily awake from a light slumber. While many people are catching Ubers home from a bar, I am getting dressed in workout attire. Excitement has replaced exhaustion. I head out the door to meet up with some fit friends at our meeting location. While it might seem a bit unorthodox to work out with little sleep, I was not alone in this adventure. Several local friends I met through Instagram were headed for South Florida for a workout meetup. This time would be very different.

The same women I did circuit training with were meeting me for a 7 a.m. beachside workout. The girls I was traveling with that day had also signed up for a Soul Cycle class afterwards. During my fitness journey, I have been following and inspired by many other "fitties" online, several of whom rave about SoulCycle. I figured it was a fad and failed to see how it was different than other cycling classes, but I was excited and ready to see what the hype was about. My first impression of the studio was energy. It may have been the girls I was with, but the vibe was electrifying before even entering the cycling room. Being surrounded by enthused people definitely makes a big impact on mood prior to exercise.

Our instructor was calm and radiated an incredible liveliness. The cycle room was dark and candle lit, a bit seductive. Upbeat music was playing and it just set the mood. It took a song or two to find my groove. I had trouble with "tapping back" while peddling fast, but the energy was so elevated, all I wanted to do was add in dance moves. It was a blast. Then came a moment that took me by completely by surprise.

We were in total darkness, the music was purely instrumental and we were peddling at a consistent pace.

Out of the blue, I found myself utterly overwhelmed with emotion; I was startled. This sensation took me by surprise -it was unexpected and just came out of nowhere. I didn't expect to become emotional; the combination of positive, dynamic energy mixed with the motivational, meditative pep talks by the instructor brought out "all the feels" in me. It was speaking directly to my soul. In that moment, I had never felt so free.

I was living in the moment. I was able to truly not think of a single thing except for being present while being able to let go, release, and allow myself to express my emotions fully. I felt mostly happiness and excitement; the overwhelming sensation was rooted in extreme joy. It was not sadness. It was an exhilaration from my soul. I was eager to learn how to hold onto that so I could have that joyfulness in my daily life.

It has been many months since that moment, and I have yet to experience it again. But I know it is there. I have felt happiness before, but not quite this extreme bliss. I am working towards adding that to my everyday life. The most beautiful thing that has emerged from my fitness journey has been self-acceptance and truly tapping into my most authentic self. My journey has been terrifying, exhilarating, and paralyzing while constantly challenging my self-awareness. I am not a very religious person, but my journey quickly became very spiritual. I began to risk and question my current life a bit more in order to find the meaning and faith I yearned for.

The next time I felt such pure and genuine happiness was Memorial Day weekend when I went to Austin. It had been a year since I decided to choose self-love over loathing, just a few days before my one-year fitness anniversary.

Through my online documentation of my story, I have connected and bonded with some pretty incredible people. In December of 2015, I flew to New York City by myself and stayed with women I had never met before. Definitely a moment where I stepped outside my comfort zone, I was so incredibly nervous and did not know what to expect. I wondered if they would like me in person, if I would be judged for not looking the way I was presented online. It was scary to navigate this big city alone. Oddly enough, I was not afraid of rooming with random women I had met online. I just trusted they were as benign and friendly as they seemed on Instagram. My very short visit to New York City will be one I cherish forever. It was an absolute blast and I would definitely have regretted not going. I played it safe though; I was a bit reserved and did not quite feel comfortable allowing myself to be completely me.

One of the women I roomed with in New York City opened her home up to a few of us during Memorial Day weekend. Two of the women were flying in from California and I considered them to be my internet best friends. I had connected with them early on in my journey and had been dying to meet them in person. It was finally happening! The trip was far too short. From the moment I met these women to the moment we said goodbye, I have never been so happy. As I said, I am not one to cry in front of others, but the moment we said goodbye I couldn't hold back the tears. They fell without hesitation and I allowed myself to just let it happen.

From the moment I met these women, I felt entirely free to be me. I didn't feel embarrassed, I didn't feel judged, I didn't feel reserved or shy. I never felt so comfortable and uninhibited. I didn't even have to ask myself, "is it ok to be weird this weekend?" because I just knew from the very first moment I met these women that I could be any way I wanted to be. I took far more ridiculous-faced pictures that weekend than normal ones. I rarely make silly faces in photos because there is a level of exposure in intentionally being unattractive. I honestly love every single "ugly" outtake picture I took on that trip. I can look at these snaps and see someone confident and comfortable in their skin, a new me! Those women did not bring out the best in me, they brought out the whole, complete, authentic, genuine, natural, imperfect, and unapologetically real me. Words can't describe how incredibly freeing it was. They laughed with me, not at me, and they completely embraced all that I am. When you can be completely confident and comfortable with your true and honest self around people you're meeting for the first time, you know you have found a truly special bond. Surround yourself with those who do not simply bring out the best in you, but allow you to be the rawest, most real, authentically genuine version of you. Learn to laugh at the perfectly imperfect and most human parts of you.

My little sister told me she envied me in high school because I spoke so confidently about "what I wanted to do and be when I grew up." She thought self-awareness was something she needed to figure out before college. She is four years younger than me, and she told me she thought she had to know her future path while still in middle school. Some people know from a very early age what they want to do and be. I thought I was one of those people, too. But as I have transformed on my journey, I have learned I didn't yet know myself. My journey has brought me closer to that realization.

My little sister now wants to join the Peace Corp after graduation. It alarms me and I have expressed my reservations about her joining. But those are my fears. She cannot live my fears. This is her dream and she needs to live it. I am a little envious of her for this incredible opportunity for self-discovery. I never had that wild and adventurous side. I never expected to find more of myself in my fitness journey. It came as a total surprise. That being said, I don't know all of me yet, but more of my truest self has been revealed. Finding and knowing yourself shouldn't ever stop. I don't think are ever "don" or "complete" as humans. I think we can always discover just a little bit more about ourselves, and that is where greatness lives, in the dark, deep corners of our most authentic selves. I don't think "finding yourself" has to go hand in hand with a fitness journey or lifestyle necessarily, but it helped me understand myself more fully. This came about from opening my heart to the energy of others.

My whole journey has not been about losing weight and exercising to achieve a certain body look. Yes, I have goals I am working towards, but my journey has very much evolved into trying to find what sets my soul on fire and determining what it truly means to be me. The very first time I did SoulCycle, I was skeptical of the hype. Yet during that first session where I was deeply moved, in that moment, I truly knew who I was and what I wanted to do. It was quite an emotional and empowering moment.

You don't have to know what you want to do or who you want to be at 16, 26, or even at 56. People change. Passions evolve. Part of knowing who you are and finding all that you are meant to become sometimes involves an unraveling of who you thought you were. It can be intimidating but so liberating. Knowing who you are is the freedom to choose to become self-aware, happy, and content with all of who you are in the present moment. You realize your worth is no longer bound by your external being, but by what you carry in your heart and contribute from your mind.

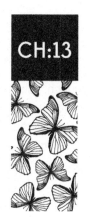

CH:13

Connected Meaning

Growing up with divorced parents, we had to split time between households: two weeks' vacation with my dad in the summertime, alternate spring breaks, Thanksgiving, and a week during the Christmas holiday. We would take weeklong vacations in summer or spend spring break at a National Park. My sister and I are big animal lovers, so we always wanted to travel where we could see wildlife or picturesque scenery. I am so thankful for this, because I found a deep love for nature and for the natural beauty of the United States. I had ups and downs on these adventures, but each vacation taught me more about myself and about life.

One year, we went to Maine, an incredibly scenic state. We headed to Acadia National Park, but when we were there, a dense fog obscured the panorama. We decided to go on a moose tour where we had the once-in-a-life time chance to see a mama moose with her calf. Late that night, we got to witness a magical moose moment. We also took in a whale

169

tour where we got to see humpback whales and a sunfish. It truly was an incredible vacation.

On that trip, I remember sitting at a restaurant for a late lunch. The restaurant was a little empty, just my family and one other party there at the time. We were sitting on the covered patio to enjoy the perfect weather. I don't remember exactly why, but the other group was really noticeable, probably a bit drunk and rowdy; I thought they were "acting weird." But we finished our meals and then went our separate ways not thinking much of it.

Every time we went on vacation, our dad started planning for the next adventure, which greatly annoyed my sister and me. I now understand all the planning that goes into a vacation, but as a child, it was far more fun to live in the moment. Our next adventure would be a visit to Yellowstone National Park.

Almost exactly a year after our trip to Maine, we were in Yellowstone hoping to see Old Faithful. It had just begun to rain, so we took refuge at the Old Faithful Lodge to wait it out. While standing around, a man walked up saying, "Hey! Weren't you guys in Maine this time last year?" We looked at one another in shock. Yes, it turns out it was the SAME man from the restaurant in Maine. What are the odds of running into a stranger across the country a year later? To this day, this memory is very vivid to me as one of the most random happenings of my life.

Another favorite vacation moment was visiting Yosemite for the first time. We were staying in Camp Curry; if you like camping and nature, it is a really nice place to unplug. While on this trip to Yosemite, we went on a stargazing tour.

We were brought to an open field where there was very little artificial light to maximize the stargazing experience. They had blankets for us, and we just laid down as the guide pointed out different constellations and told stories about the stars. It was mind-boggling yet oddly comforting. We were in a large group but it was quiet and relaxing. In that moment I felt so content and at peace and pondered many different things. I remember this as being an all-consuming and powerful experience.

You may well be wondering at this point, "Ummm, Jess, but what does any of this have to do with fitness, a healthy lifestyle, and body positivity?" And my answer is simple: It is all about being exposed and open to growth. Running into that stranger in both Maine and Yellowstone at the same exact time and same exact place cannot be purely coincidental. There is connection there. Although I may never fully understand the meaning of it, there is some reason why it happened. I learned a lot from those trips around the country. And as I continue on my fitness journey, it all blends into one big soulful, revelatory adventure.

The quest for meaning and connection was what brought me back into therapy. I had been on my journey for eight months and was feeling better about myself than ever before, but something was still missing. I was connecting with and empowering so many women to learn to love themselves, yet I still did not completely love myself. I was not sure if it was me or my life in general. I realized the connections were ultimately lacking in meaning for my life. I was being vulnerable and putting myself out there, yet the missing part was that I was not yet connected with my truest self.

I did not set out to understand or find "the meaning of life"; instead I was looking for how I could make my life more meaningful. All the relationships in my life were less successful than they could have been because I was not fully open, honest, and vulnerable in my thoughts, actions, and emotions. I didn't communicate effectively for the same reasons. My relationship with my dad suffered from this. I took everything personally and blamed both of us for our lack of connection.

The only person who I feel as though I can be my real self with is my sister. The bond we share is something I want to have in all my relationships. My way of hiding feelings is to close up and not reach out to others. I do that to this day when insecurities get the best of me. Of course, this breaks connections. As I have become older, I have worked on my relationship with my dad. I have learned that it really was all about learning to be in tune with my truest and most authentic self; this allowed me to begin healing from how I hurt myself in the past because of my perceptions of how others treated me. I always thought something wrong with me, and that I was unlikeable. I always thought I was unworthy because I was weird or different or uncool, when all I really needed to do was accept myself.

I never anticipated becoming so open and vulnerable on my fitness Instagram. Strangely, I don't view posting my "before" pictures as me being vulnerable, even though most people are too embarrassed to do so. My body is not what makes me, me. It is my inner being; WHO I am that is what makes me an individual. The vulnerability in opening up and sharing the WHO is far more intimidating than showing the WHAT. I will post an "unflattering" picture any day, because I now understand that for me, that is not vulnerability. My physicality is not what creates the meaning and connection in my life. Sharing my mind and heart, THAT is where my connection comes from. My truth, my real self, has nothing to do with appearances. For others, that may be the case, but not for me. I am able to have meaningful and connected relationships because I have a mind and heart that allow me to think, feel, and express myself. My body is simply a harbor, a home for my soul to live.

My journey took an unexpected turn from where I began. It started with the intention to become healthier and happier, which I thought would come from changing my outer appearances. Although my journey to being the healthiest and fittest version of myself is still about physical change, I recognize there is much more to it. When it comes to my body, insecurities and negative thoughts still exist. That is still only a part of the whole, which is a full experience involving mind, body, heart, and soul. To be connected and live with meaning starts with self-acceptance, inclusive of your body. Acceptance needs to begin NOW. You can like, love, and accept yourself while still working towards becoming your best self. Self-betterment involves exposure and allowing all of yourself to be seen; the good, bad, and ugly.

But for me to allow myself to be fully seen, I need to shed the metaphorical "cover up" of insecurities, doubts, and fears. I have a much more positive mindset about my body now than ever before, but that does not mean I am not without negative moments at times. This journey has been very much a roller-coaster ride. People will always judge, criticize, or put you down because your methods or beliefs are different. But you must be strong in WHO you ARE to not let this affect you and not let it define your worth and make you put that "cover up" back on. There can be negative and positive effects to a weight management journey. People will try to tell you how you should look or what your goals to achieve should be, but you must remain true to what you want to become. YOUR worth, YOUR meaning, YOUR connections should be designed by you and only you. No one could or should craft and design the vision of your soul. Only you can do that.

By putting yourself out there online, you open yourself to opinions and expectations from others. I get comments along the lines of, "You are the perfect amount of softness," "You are a real woman because you have curves,""You do not need to change anymore." While these are meant to be kind comments, they still reflect some societal pressure telling me what I should look like, even though I strive not to base my worth on my appearance and what others think of me. The whole problem with body insecurities are the messed up "beauty standards" telling us who we should be, what we should do, how we should act, and what we should look like as women.

Personally, I do not like hearing women being classified and defined as "real" solely because they look a certain way. I am not any more real because I have curves. I am real because I am human. I am real because I have thoughts, experiences, and emotions. I'm no more or less real than anyone else. A woman is no less feminine if she is thin or more muscular. A girl is no less attractive whether she is bigger or a little curvier. The only true "realness" is that I am learning to become unapologetically me. Every BODY is different and there is beauty in that! REAL is not skinny, or fat, or thick, or curvy, or muscular. These descriptive words should not be used to describe a "real woman." Real is so much deeper than that. Real is emotion, character, personality. Real lies within your heart and mind, because that's where the WHO translates to the YOU that is shared with the world. The only realness to me is that I choose to be no one else but me. Being real is honestly so comforting and freeing because I feel like I don't have to force my body into looking a certain way. Embracing myself as I am today takes the increasing pressure of expectations away. Its helps me let go of the pressure of what I feel I should be and look like based on society's standards projected onto all females. The only standard I have to meet is the one I set for myself, and there is nothing more liberating than being true to my heart and mind. Being emotionally and consciously vulnerable has allowed my soul to become free from the imprisonment of my body so that I can create a meaningful life with the connectedness I desire.

I am still in therapy trying to figure out what this meaning is for me so that I can begin making the connections in life that I desire. I have lots of ideas as to what they are, but there still much that remains unknown. Once I can connect with and help both girls and women become their truest selves, living freely with the body confidence they deserve, only then will I be living with meaning. By helping other women feel empowerment, self-love, and respect of themselves and others, it will all be worth it to open myself up in sharing my story. What I have shared is just a fraction of my life and the growing confidence that has manifested within the last year. I can tell you there is no greater gift you can give yourself than learning to love who you are or who you are becoming. It is not vain to love yourself; it is not pompous or conceited. It might seem defiant given that society emphasizes self-disgust based on unrealistic standards. Self-love is necessary. Self-love is deserved. Self-love is important.

My growing body-positive confidence comes from many places. I no longer look at other women and girls with my "goal body" in mind. I look at them in admiration for the hard work they have put into improving themselves. I used to compare and body-shame others in some sad attempt to feel better about myself. I'm grateful I no longer do that, because it's simply unkind. If I catch myself doing that, I stop myself immediately.

I don't know what path any other woman has walked or the insecurities she deals with. I don't know the doubts, fears, or negative thoughts that may weigh down her mind. I now look at her with compassion and the understanding that she has battles and struggles she's working through, because we ALL do. I no longer see others for what their body shape or size is. I see others as people, not bodies. I see their hearts and souls and personality and the special spark that makes them uniquely beautiful. I've been able to adopt this mindset because I've learned to see myself this way. I don't define myself by what my body is or is not, I define myself by how I treat others and myself and who I'm becoming as an individual. My body has changed, but so has my heart and mind. And that's been the biggest reward of all. We CAN redefine unrealistic ideals of body image and societal standards. It starts with you. It starts with me. It starts with her, she, and WE! Women HAVE to stop putting other women down. We need to be a united front so that we can continue to fight for and strive for equality and change unrealistic standards of beauty. We all have this greatest gift in common: we are living a HUMAN experience, not a perfect one. Humans are far from perfect. Our imperfections make us human.

A more meaningful and connected human experience should be less focused on the visual. It should be felt, expressed, thought; emotional and spiritual. Your brain is your most powerful tool; use that power wisely to spread joy, happiness, kindness, and positivity. Looks and beauty will always be subjective and they fade over time anyway. Your thoughts, actions, language, and the way you spread and show love are more powerful, energizing, and longer lasting. I will always strive to put inner beauty before outer, because life is fragile. Life is too short to let a few body imperfections define our worth and control our feelings of "enough-ness." We are all the same, in that we all share a thinking mind and beating heart. Each of us is unique, of course, but the same power is within all of us. How you chose to use that power is up to you.

We live in a fast-paced world where we want immediate gratification and results. To craft a meaningful life spent pursuing your passions, you need to understand that it takes time. And as my mom says, "Time takes time." You can live the life you have always dreamed, but it will not happen by watching, wishing, or complaining. It happens with patience, action, and doing. Don't rush your progress with either body confidence or cultivating a life you can take pride in.

Don't rush the process, either. If you do, you are essentially rushing your life. You will miss out on YOUR very real, human, and vulnerable experiences, because you will become too focused on becoming what others want you to be. You risk missing out on understanding the truth of who you really are. Living happily and healthily truly is a LIFEstyle. The best way to live it is in the manner that works and feels right for you. It can change as you adapt and grow. Change is part of the process. If nothing changes, we are not growing. Do no limit your potential. Constantly question yourself in a positive manner that allows you to flourish. Become confident in WHO you are by continuously proving yourself wrong. Break the barriers of self-imprisonment from bodily insecurities that hinders your soul from being not just touched with light, but seen with grace.

The meanings and connections we make in life are so much deeper than our ephemeral beings. Both meeting the stranger in Yellowstone and stargazing in Yosemite reminded me just how big the universe is, yet how small our world can be. Life is too short not to live a life you are proud to live, happy with, and created just for you as you see it. You CAN achieve anything you set your mind to. Whether you want to change your body or change the course of your life, you need to believe in yourself, have faith, and chase that dream with vigor, passion, and positivity. It is possible. You CAN live a life free of body insecurities. It begins with a little understanding of who you are and focusing on establishing a healthy mind and happy heart. Self-love begins withIN you. Understand that this does not happen overnight. It happens over time. That is the beauty in the journey. But to enjoy the destination, you must remember to love yourself every step of the way. What is stopping you from loving yourself today?

Live your truest, most authentic, and most real human experience unbound by insecurities; only then can your soul be set free of self-imprisonment and judgment. You are worth fighting for. You are worthy of allowing your soul to shine!

Thank you for trusting, believing, and being interested in my "average yet real "story. Thank you for not criticizing or judging my insecurities. Thank you for allowing me to be weak. Thank you for allowing me to be human.

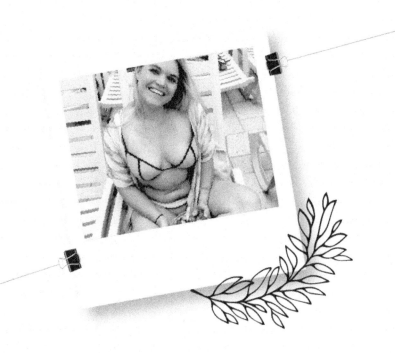

CH:14

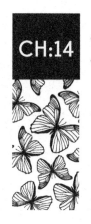

Designing Your Body Positive Masterpiece

As I have mentioned before, I am not a therapist or expert in body positivity. I really am just a regular girl on my own journey sharing my story, thoughts, and how I changed my mindset along the way. What has worked for me might not work for you, but if I can help just one girl or woman feel better about herself, more confident, and less focused on what her body looks like, I will be happy. The interactive activities included in this book are solely to be utilized as tools to challenge how you view yourself. Everything is simply a suggestion and something I have learned on my journey that hopefully can be integrated as new knowledge into thinking a little differently. Every woman I follow online expresses observations from their journey and transformation of their MIND. I really and truly believe that to succeed in changing both your body and life, you need to start with the right mindset.

In the same way thatwe build and strengthen our body, our mind needs to be conditioned to delete negativity and allow positivity in. My brain is a muscle I am constantly working to strengthen as negativity seeps into my mind at times of weakness. I have now conditioned my brain in such a way that the negativity that comes in is rarely about my body or how I feel about myself; the negativity takes on a deeper meaning and is more about finding the lost connections and meaning in my life. This is something I have striven to point out, not letting the negativity overtake my emotional disposition. We must cultivate a mind filled with positive thoughts, a garden for growth. There will be pests of negativity, but we must find the right thoughts to question the internalized messages that adversely affect our mindset and emotions.

A strong body is so much more than physical and a visual expression. We need to end the judgments we place upon ourselves and no longer endure living in self-destruction. We must challenge ourselves to growth, exposure, and renewal, over and over again to fully flourish and bloom. The strength we manifest and possess should live and thrive from within. Our bodies are nothing more than a home for who we were and who we are to become. Our bodies are our unspoken stories; we can never rewrite a past chapter, but we can always shape the one we are in. It is SO important to grow your mind and harbor the positive thoughts and feelings that feel right for you.

I carried weight around for many years, both literally and figuratively, and used it as a cushion to conceal my emotions. My moments of negativity ebb and flow like the tide when I'm in a trying period of self-doubt. But instead of focusing on the fact that I don't have the flattest stomach or most defined legs and arms, I'm focusing on what my body IS and DOES for me. I have a body that allows me to do the things I love! First and foremost, it allows me to be expressive, creative, and BE uniquely me – I get to be an individual because my body is different and no one else can ever have it. There is beauty in that, and my body also allows me to walk, run, jump, swim, bike, do push-ups, and DANCE. It allows me to think, converse, connect, and have a voice. Beauty is subjective, much like art. Everyone has their different preferences. I have a strong art background, and I think all art is interesting and beautiful in its own unique way, despite how diverse it may be. And I have realized there is ART to the HUMAN form. You are the artist to YOUR life. You can imagine and create it any way you want. Your body is YOUR masterpiece. Draw it, paint it, sculpt it, and create it with care. There is beauty in creating a life and body that is YOUR vision; there is power in that you are uniquely YOU. You are the best project you'll ever work on, so never stop constructing your masterpiece.

How do you design a body-positive masterpiece? I genuinely believe it begins with nourishing the body, mind, heart, and soul together as a whole being. It is important to recognize and understand our weaknesses so that we can reinforce them to strengthen our whole human experience. There are tough questions that must be asked and answered. This chapter is interactive, and my intention is that it brings out your best thoughts and ideas for selfie love with journaling prompts, things to ponder, and things to challenge yourself. Think of these tools as symbolic "gym bag essentials" for your whole being. They are just meant to make you think a little bit and challenge your mindset so that you can really and fully comprehend how you see yourself and how you can change in a positive manner!

I had to build my self-esteem alone. Maybe I didn't have to, but that is certainly how it began. I had to figure out how to love myself, because no one can do that for you. I was in a place where I could not yet find that self-love. This book is not intended to replace a therapist or life coach's services; I cannot guarantee it will help. Think of it more as a guide for your own efforts, a starting point to allow you to question your inner dialogue and being. Hopefully, it will spark you to create questions to challenge yourself on your journey. Again, these are questions I have had to ask myself about my body negativity. There is no right or wrong way to do this; just allow yourself to question where the pessimism comes from. But if you do not do this work, you will avoid discovering the deep roots of your insecurity-driven thoughts. I didn't arrive at my increased confidence and improved body-positive mindset by evading my feelings. I did that long enough in the past. I had to actually allow myself to go to a place of serious discomfort; in many ways I still have to do this. I harbored the notion of being a "victim of circumstance" for far too long; I did this by avoiding facing my feelings. I used my body as a metaphorical shield to hide those limiting beliefs and keep my soul sheltered. It was not by shedding weight that I to found myself, it was by no longer avoiding my thoughts, feelings, and emotions. I believe that to begin to create a healthy self-image, you must go to that place of discomfort. I allowed my anxieties and fears to keep me from trying for too long. Hesitation and fear of trying created an even worse self-image. In my journey, I found it was better to at least try and see what I was capable of, because I often surprised myself. Even if I didn't succeed, I began to feel better simply because I put effort in and gave it my all. Staying on the safe side and not facing fears might seem more comfortable, but it is in actuality the opposite. You risk avoiding realizing your fullest potential because you allow your fears and anxieties to rule instead of learning how to prove yourself wrong by challenging those fears. Confronting my anxiety, fears, and doubts has only contributed to a growing sense of worth, confidence, esteem, and self-love. I hope the following questions can help you begin to question and fight your own inner demons a little more. Time to get a little uncomfortable!

Nourishment

Nourish the Body

- First and foremost, do your research. Learn about new and exciting ways to be active and explore those options and discover what is not just challenging but fun for you. Also, educate yourself on proper nutrition. You do not have to be an expert to be a success. Success comes with trial and error and allowing yourself to fail. That way, you continuously learn.

- What is your WHY for wanting to get into shape or live a healthy lifestyle? Your why must be for the right reasons so that this is not simply a short-lived fad and can become your lifestyle. Your why can be your motivation. But in terms of motivation, there are some things to keep in mind. Are you externally and negatively-influenced (I want to change my body so that I can find love and a significant other)? Or are you internally negatively- influenced (I want to lose weight so that I love myself)? If yes, how can you be positively influenced to want to start living a healthier lifestyle? For me, once I stopped feeling that I had to lose weight to be attractive or worthy and focused on wanting to lose weight to be healthier because my body deserved it, my motivation stuck!

- What is one thing you can do less of that is an unhealthy habit?

- What is one thing you can do more of that is a healthier habit?

- Pick a day of the week to set your weekly goals and stick to that plan.

- Do something simple such as prepping your meals for the next day. You do not have to have it all figured out and prepare a week's worth of macro-friendly meals if you are new to this lifestyle. Start with small and manageable things you can do.

- What are your long-term fitness goals?

- What are some short-term fitness goals?

- Are all your goals based on visual changes to your body? If so, how can you craft some new goals that focus on other values, whether they are strength, exercise, or even life-based?

- Maybe you are a busy mom, or a student, or a career woman, how can you make YOU a priority? What is most important for YOU to maintain your body's health?

- What is one thing you love about your body today? Can't find anything? There is something you MUST love! If you cannot find something on your body, how about something you love in who you ARE?

- What is one thing you are thankful for that your body does for you?

- Maybe loving your body is tough today; how can you learn to love your body?

- What do you think being pretty or skinny will accomplish, if that is your main focus behind losing weight?

  - What will that bring to your life? Do you think it will add value and happiness?

  - What are other ways you can channel value and happiness into your life that go beyond your body's appearance?

Nourish the Mind

- Look in the mirror. What do you SEE? Analyze all of you. What are your thoughts? What do you FEEL? Are they happy, or sad, or angry, or frustrated? Is what you see and feel positive or negative? If negative, in what ways can you change your mindset? What would need to change for you to see yourself in a positive manner?

- Name all the things you love about yourself.

  - How many of these things are related to your body?

  - How many of these things are related to your personality and who you are?

- Do you still compare yourself to others? Do you look at other women and think, "I want to be her" or "I want her body"? WHY?

  - If yes, how can you stop comparing? What will make you feel better about yourself that is isolated from other's appearances or life?

- What is your biggest insecurity in both body and personality (perhaps you wish you were not so shy)? In what ways can you begin to change these things you feel you must "cover up"?

- Do you define yourself in terms of numbers? Does the number on the scale define your happiness and contentment? Why do you place so much emphasis on that number, or on any number for that matter? Remember, the scale, pants size, waist size, bust size, and all the rest are simply units of measurement. They should be utilized as data points, not as a way to define your worth.

- What are your limiting beliefs about who you are?

- What is mindfulness to you? And how can you be more mindful throughout the day?

- What is presence to you? And how can you be more emotionally, mentally, and physically present?

- Try not to focus so much on being motivated. I often get asked how I stay motivated, but it is not so much motivation for me, but simply that this lifestyle is not just a habit, but now my new normal. Both bad habits and good habits can be easy to establish and maintain. Think of your bad habits. Think of your good habits. What good habits do you feel you are lacking? What bad habits can you release?

- Do you tend to be an "energy sucker" with your negative mindset? I find when I am surrounded by people with negative energy that it brings me down. Maybe you cannot always control your surroundings or environment, but you can foster an environment inside you that is protected from that negativity. What positive thoughts can you cultivate to guard against the negative energies of others?

- Why do we allow others to dictate our emotions and feelings so much? Even someone who is a total stranger? I recently had a guy cut me off on the road, risking danger to everyone around. I fumed for hours afterwards – why were his needs more important than mine? I allowed the situation to consume and bother me for the rest of the day. Why could I not just let go and release? How can you learn to allow yourself to release and let go? When you fall mentally, emotionally, or physically,

189

how will you get back up? The need that propels us to keep moving forward is the momentum needed to get back up and stay on track.

°   What thoughts, feelings, and emotions are you avoiding feeling? How can you allow yourself to feel them?

Nourish the Heart

Listen to the tone of voice you use when you speak to yourself. Is it harsh? Is it kind? Is it ia tone you would use to speak to others you love and care about?

How do you want others to think of you and speak about you?

When you think of the comforts of home, what comes to mind? How can you gather those feelings within your own heart?

To find comfort within a healthy and self-loving heart, you have to get to that place, and it might not be easy. There may be pain associated with self-reflection; are you afraid to analyze yourself too much? To be able to remove fear and doubt from your heart, you must find where they hide deep inside.

Think of how you love and feel for others. How can you establish that feeling within yourself?

Ask others, close friends and family, how they see you, how they think about you, how they feel about you. This may well be uncomfortable, but to understand

Designing Your Body Positive Masterpiece

how others SEE you might help you see yourself a little differently. I have known for a long time how my little sister sees me in a positive light, but it took me so long to see myself in the same manner. What is it you may be holding on to that keeps you from seeing yourself in the light of others?

Write a letter to your younger self. What do you say? What do you feel? How do you let go of what was so that you can embrace what is?

Write a a letter to your daughter, or future daughter, or younger sister, or niece or any little girl in your life who is important to you. What are the things you want her to know and value in herself so that she can learn that self-love and respect are not just acceptable, but necessary?

Nourish the Soul

- What makes you feel "seen?"

- Do you like feeling invisible? Why?

- Do you feel you are lacking meaning and connection in your life? What do meaning and connection feel and look like for you? How can you change your current situation to achieve living with more purpose?

- Sadly, some people are shallow and only see you for what you look like. I have learned that to see true beauty, look deeply within others to know WHO they are inside. That is what matters, not

191

WHAT they look like. Always remember you are more than a body. You are beautiful because your soul is so very unique. What can you keep in mind when someone judges or disapproves of your appearance so that you remain true to your soul?

○ What does confidence look like to you? How can you create that vision within yourself?

○ Do a daily reflection and a daily check-in with yourself. This can be done in writing or simply by contemplating your thoughts internally.

○ Sometimes when we are in the process of self-discovery, we can get caught up in comparing our old self to our new self. You can feel trapped in a body or mind that once was. In what ways can you let go of the "old" or "younger" you so that you can embrace the new?

○ It is easy to get caught up in comparing not just your body but your life to others' and wanting to vicariously live through other people who either seem to "have it all together" or have a more adventurous and fun-filled life than yours. What is the dream you have for YOUR life? Can you visualize where you want to be? Maybe you are there, or where you thought you wanted to be, yet something doesn't feel right or is missing. What would make you feel more fulfilled? How will you work towards achieving that?

○ I might not have a daughter yet, but I do have a younger sister. Sometimes we get so absorbed in our own problems that we forget who is watching. Someone in your life will be watching. Do you want them to see the overanalysis and unkindness? Do you want them to learn to become obsessed with and valued only for what their bodies look like? Or do you want her to learn respect, care, kindness, and love towards for herself as well as for others? How can you treat yourself more kindly so that they learn to treat themselves in a similar way?

° Your story, your thoughts, your feelings, your being are so very important. You are worthy of being shared with the world. How will you begin to start sharing yourself?

° What is stopping you from allowing your soul to shine?

Conclusion

You are a unique individual, not a standard.

This past year has been a year of self-awakening. Although I started out my journey wanting to be happier and healthier and thinking that losing weight would do the trick, I have realized that happiness, confidence, self-worth, and love can be achieved regardless of what my body looks like. Don't get me wrong, there are still days I wake up and wish I looked different or felt prettier. There are many days I wished I could lose fat faster and change my body quicker. However, I found that my growing worth and confidence is in recognizing that *who* I am has changed. Yes my looks are changing, but so is my heart and soul. Being willing to wear a bikini shows confidence, but that does not mean I do so without insecurities or hesitation. Confidence, for me, is being brave with allowing my true self to shine. What I hope you take away from all this is that confidence is loving *who* you are and not letting what you look like define your whole being.

I don't want you to think that body positivity is always constant. It ebbs and flows with the good and bad moments. But that's what makes it a journey. This journey that I have shared is yours now. Learn from it, grow from it and find your happiness.

I understand body confidence is very challenging, especially in today's society where unrealistic standards are admired even though they are almost impossible to meet. I posed the question on my Instagram asking what biggest factors are that contribute to each of your struggles with a body positive mindset. The responses were very congruent with many of the stories I have shared in this book:

- perfectionism
- feelings of inadequacy
- lack of confidence
- not fitting the mold of societal standards
- a flawed reflection in the mirror
- the fashion and clothing industry
- pressure
- failure
- comparison to others

My initial response to all of this is FUCK.BEAUTY. STANDARDS.

You are a unique individual, not a standard. I know we live in a day and age when we feel like we have to fit into some cookie cutter mold. But where is the character and vibrancy in that? Always remember there is an offline to an online. Sure, a girl you see online might appear to be your idea of a perfect example of "body goals" but you still don't know what path she walked to get there, or what struggles she had or still has with self-acceptance. I see women skinnier than me who still struggle with being content in their own skin. It reminds me that body dissatisfaction does NOT discriminate on shape or size. We all struggle with something. We all struggle differently.

Beauty is such a tricky thing; we are visual beings. But understand that looks do fade, and your body may abandon you one day. But even if your body does not function "normally," you are still beautiful if you practice cultivating a beautiful mind, heart, and soul.

You must allow yourself to thaw. Warm up to the ideas, concepts, and perceptions that you are enough, you are worthy, you are beautiful TODAY. Thaw out the struggles, insecurities, doubts and fears. The separation. The breaking. The exit. The reveal. The thaw. It will allow you to find a sense of home within.

To thaw is to be open, connected, vulnerable, emotionally intimate, and truthful. To warm is to expand and break, to make room and fill the void with purpose, passion, and meaning. Don't thaw into the idea of wanting to know all of you, warm into the reveal of the discovery of becoming who you were meant to become all along. Leave your winter and find your spring. Honor these seasons; thaw with grace, and grow with dignity. Thaw your hardened, sad, and negative heart so that your mind can grow, expand, and embrace the self-love you deserve.

You must allow yourself to heal. It is not about healing the physical and changing your body. It is about healing those dark places in both heart and mind, bringing the light in and letting the warmth release them from cold despair. Heal from the negative self-talk. Heal into self-discovery that is neither bound nor limited by an exterior shell. Heal into your truest most authentic self. Heal into who you are yet to become. You are not becoming a more desirable body, you are on your way to becoming a more valuable human. Humans are flawed and imperfect, so why strive for "perfection"? Heal *with* your flaws and imperfections. Do not heal because of them or as a way to spite them. Heal with your heart, mind, and soul first, then your inner dialogue on how you see your physical self will begin to change. You won't be looking at fat and cellulite and rolls, you will be looking at a kinder and gentler heart, a stronger and wiser mind, and a confident and undeniably beautiful soul.

When we care for ourselves from a place of self-love, appreciation, and respect, we can more easily act upon our beautiful purpose and live a very real and HUMAN experience. Beauty should no longer be a cerebral expectation constructed by societal beliefs. Beauty is choosing to live our own unique story that is not merely ephemeral existence, but a harmonized story created in our bodies and hearts, our very real and human story. You are not perfect. You are not a number. You are not a failure. You are not fat or ugly or unworthy. You are not your genetics. You are not her. You are you.

You are enough. You are complete. You are living your human experience. Now go live fully, freely, and unbound by your body so you can let your happy heart and confident soul shine!

Acknowledgments

I would like to thank my mentor for being there for me through the whole process of writing this book. Writing this has opened old wounds. while also healing some scars and causing me to question many things from my past. Her understanding and truly knowing me better than anyone else gave me the confidence to pursue this project with passion and belief in myself. I have grown with her guidance through this process. She helped me and encouraged me to share my story while reminding me that it is just that: my experience, my story.

I sincerely thank anyone who has been a part of my journey, either from the beginning or more recently. Every one of you has contributed to my growth and better understanding of myself. Without your support and encouragement, I would have missed out on this great gift of knowing me. The stories that you share and your openness in allowing me into not just your lives but your hearts enriches my life; you let me know I am not alone and remind me that we are all struggling, but now we struggle together. You all have impacted me and touched me in some way. Thank you for being a part of my story!

Author Bio

Jessica Pack is a certified life coach striving to help young girls and women feel comfortable in the skin they are in today. She shares her fitness journey in the hope that it may encourage women and girls to see the beauty in who they are, while challenging the constraints of poor body image issues that often lead to feelings of unworthiness and of never being enough. Her raw, relatable, and vulnerable story captivates as she shares how she abandoned poor body image and embraced self-love, acceptance, and worth. Her mission is to help girls and women feel comfortable accepting that it is okay to be imperfectly beautiful, because at the end of the day, we are all the same: human!

Jessica Pack

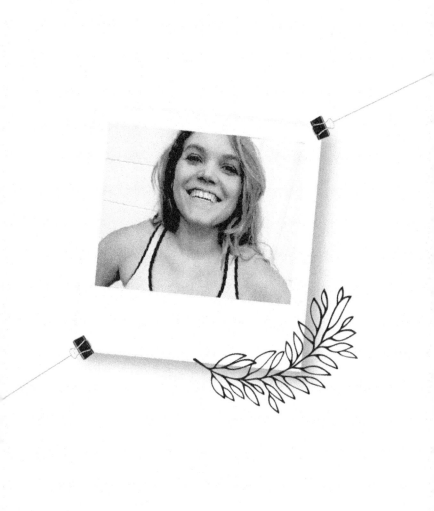

CPSIA information can be obtained
at www.ICGtesting.com
Printed in the USA
BVOW03s0025281116
468953BV00003B/3/P